Minimally Invasive Neonatal Surgery

Editors

MARK L. WULKAN
HANMIN LEE

CLINICS IN PERINATOLOGY

www.perinatology.theclinics.com

Consulting Editor
LUCKY JAIN

December 2017 • Volume 44 • Number 4

ELSEVIER

1600 John F. Kennedy Boulevard • Suite 1800 • Philadelphia, Pennsylvania, 19103-2899

http://www.theclinics.com

CLINICS IN PERINATOLOGY Volume 44, Number 4
December 2017 ISSN 0095-5108, ISBN-13: 978-0-323-55292-9

Editor: Kerry Holland
Developmental Editor: Casey Potter

Clinics in Perinatology (ISSN 0095-5108) is published quarterly by Elsevier Inc., 360 Park Avenue South, New York, NY 10010-1710. Months of issue are March, June, September, and December. Business and Editorial Offices: 1600 John F. Kennedy Blvd., Ste. 1800, Philadelphia, PA 19103-2899. Customer Service Office: 3251 Riverport Lane, Maryland Heights, MO 63043. Periodicals postage paid at New York, NY and additional mailing offices. Subscription prices are $299.00 per year (US individuals), $532.00 per year (US institutions), $350.00 per year (Canadian individuals), $651.00 per year (Canadian institutions), $433.00 per year (international individuals), $651.00 per year (international institutions), $100.00 per year (US students), and $195.00 per year (Canadian and international students). International air speed delivery is included in all Clinics subscription prices. All prices are subject to change without notice. **POSTMASTER:** Send address changes to *Clinics in Perinatology*, Elsevier Health Sciences Division, Subscription Customer Service, 3251 Riverport Lane, Maryland Heights, MO 63043. **Customer Service: Telephone: 1-800-654-2452** (U.S. and Canada); **1-314-447-8871** (outside U.S. and Canada). **Fax: 1-314-447-8029. E-mail: journalscustomerservice-usa@elsevier.com** (for print support); **journalsonlinesupport-usa@elsevier.com** (for online support).

Reprints. For copies of 100 or more, of articles in this publication, please contact the Commercial Reprints Department, Elsevier Inc., 360 Park Avenue South, New York, NY 10010-1710. Tel. 212-633-3874; Fax: 212-633-3820; E-mail: reprints@elsevier.com.

Clinics in Perinatology is also pubilshed in Spanish by McGraw-Hill Interamericana Editores S.A., P.O. Box 5-237, 06500 Mexico D.F., Mexico.

Clinics in Perinatology is covered in *MEDLINE/PubMed (Index Medicus) Current Contents, Excepta Medica, BIOSIS and ISI/BIOMED.*

Printed in the United States of America.

Contributors

CONSULTING EDITOR

LUCKY JAIN, MD, MBA
Richard W. Blumberg Professor and Interim Chair, Emory University School of Medicine, Department of Pediatrics, Executive Medical Director and Interim Chief Academic Officer, Children's Healthcare of Atlanta, Atlanta, Georgia, USA

EDITORS

MARK L. WULKAN, MD, FACS, FAAP
Surgeon-in-Chief, Professor of Surgery and Pediatrics, Department of Surgery, Division of Pediatric Surgery, Children's Healthcare of Atlanta, Emory University School of Medicine, Atlanta, Georgia, USA

HANMIN LEE, MD
Surgeon in Chief, UCSF Benioff Children's Hospital, Vice Chair, Department of Surgery, Division of Pediatric Surgery, University of California San Francisco, San Francisco, California, USA

AUTHORS

SOPHIA ABDULHAI, MD
Research Fellow, Division of Pediatric Surgery, Akron Children's Hospital, Akron, Ohio, USA

SARAH B. CAIRO, MD, MPH
Pediatric Surgery Research Fellow, Department of Pediatric Surgery, Women & Children's Hospital of Buffalo, Buffalo, New York, USA

SUJIT K. CHOWDHARY, MCh, FRCS
Director, Pediatric Urology and Pediatric Surgery, Apollo Institute of Pediatric Sciences, New Delhi, India

MATTHEW S. CLIFTON, MD, FACS, FAAP
Associate Professor of Surgery and Pediatrics, Department of Surgery, Division of Pediatric Surgery, Emory University School of Medicine, Atlanta, Georgia, USA

ALEJANDRO V. GARCIA, MD, FAAP
Associate Professor, Department of Surgery, Division of Pediatric Surgery, Johns Hopkins University, Baltimore, Maryland, USA

IAN C. GLENN, MD
Research Fellow, Division of Pediatric Surgery, Akron Children's Hospital, Akron, Ohio, USA

CLAIRE E. GRAVES, MD
Postdoctoral Research Fellow, Department of Surgery, University of California San Francisco, San Francisco, California, USA

CARROLL M. HARMON, MD, PhD
John E. Fisher Chair in Pediatric Surgery, Chief, Division of Pediatric Surgery, Women & Children's Hospital of Buffalo, Program Director, Pediatric Surgery Fellowship Program, Associate Professor, Department of Surgery, The State University of New York, University at Buffalo, Buffalo, New York, USA

MICHAEL R. HARRISON, MD
Professor Emeritus of Surgery, Pediatrics, Obstetrics, Gynecology, and Reproductive Sciences, University of California San Francisco, San Francisco, California, USA

CAROLINE C.C. HULSKER, MD
Pediatric Surgeon, Department of Pediatric Surgery, University Medical Center Utrecht, Utrecht, The Netherlands

HANMIN LEE, MD
Surgeon in Chief, UCSF Benioff Children's Hospital, Vice Chair, Department of Surgery, Division of Pediatric Surgery, University of California San Francisco, San Francisco, California, USA

JEFFREY LUKISH, MD, FACS
Associate Professor, Department of Surgery, Division of Pediatric Surgery, Johns Hopkins University, Baltimore, Maryland, USA

OMID MADADI-SANJANI, MD
Centre of Pediatric Surgery Hannover, Hannover Medical School, Hannover, Germany

GO MIYANO, MD, PhD
Associate Professor, Department of Pediatric Surgery, Juntendo University School of Medicine, Tokyo, Japan

JARRETT MOYER, MD
Resident, Department of Surgery, University of California San Francisco, San Francisco, California, USA

BENJAMIN E. PADILLA, MD
Assistant Professor, Department of Surgery, Division of Pediatric Surgery, University of California San Francisco, San Francisco, California, USA

CLAUS PETERSEN, PhD
Centre of Pediatric Surgery Hannover, Hannover Medical School, Hannover, Germany

TODD A. PONSKY, MD
Associate Professor of Surgery and Pediatrics, Division of Pediatric Surgery, Akron Children's Hospital, Akron, Ohio, USA

STEVEN S. ROTHENBERG, MD
Pediatric Surgery, Rocky Mountain Hospital for Children, Denver, Colorado, USA

DAVID H. ROTHSTEIN, MD, MS
Pediatric Surgeon, Department of Pediatric Surgery, Women & Children's Hospital of Buffalo, Associate Professor, Department of Surgery, The State University of New York, University at Buffalo, Buffalo, New York, USA

BETHANY J. SLATER, MD
Pediatric Surgery, Rocky Mountain Hospital for Children, Denver, Colorado, USA

BIJI SREEDHAR, PhD
Visiting Research Fellow, School of Biomedical Sciences, Faculty of Medicine, The Chinese University of Hong Kong, Shatin, New Territories, Hong Kong

MASAHIRO TAKEDA, MD, PhD
Assistant Professor, Department of Pediatric Surgery, Juntendo University School of Medicine, Tokyo, Japan

STEFAAN H.A. TYTGAT, MD, PhD
Pediatric Surgeon, Department of Pediatric Surgery, University Medical Center Utrecht, Utrecht, The Netherlands

BENNO URE, PhD
Centre of Pediatric Surgery Hannover, Hannover Medical School, Hannover, Germany

DAVID C. VAN DER ZEE, MD, PhD
Professor, Department of Pediatric Surgery, University Medical Center Utrecht, Utrecht, The Netherlands

MAUD Y.A. VAN HERWAARDEN, MD, PhD
Pediatric Surgeon, Department of Pediatric Surgery, University Medical Center Utrecht, Utrecht, The Netherlands

LAN VU, MD
Assistant Professor, Department of Surgery, Division of Pediatric Surgery, University of California San Francisco, San Francisco, California, USA

MARIEKE J. WITVLIET, MD
Pediatric Surgeon, Department of Pediatric Surgery, University Medical Center Utrecht, Utrecht, The Netherlands

MARK L. WULKAN, MD, FACS, FAAP
Surgeon-in-Chief, Professor of Surgery and Pediatrics, Department of Surgery, Division of Pediatric Surgery, Children's Healthcare of Atlanta, Emory University School of Medicine, Atlanta, Georgia, USA

ATSUYUKI YAMATAKA, MD, PhD, FAAP (Hon)
Professor, Department of Pediatric Surgery, Juntendo University School of Medicine, Tokyo, Japan

CHUNG-KWONG YEUNG, MD, PhD, FRCS, FRACS, FACS
Honorary Clinical Professor, Department of Surgery, The University of Hong Kong, Pokfulam, Hong Kong

Contents

Imperforate anus, a variant of anorectal malformation (ARM), is a common congenital anomaly requiring surgical attention in the newborn period. It may present with a variety of anatomic configurations, largely dependent on the presence and location of a fistula. The location (or characteristics) of a fistula, which usually lies between the gastrointestinal tract and the genitourinary tract or perineum, is often used in determining the type and timing of operative management. This article discusses the work-up and management, modes of treatment and their postoperative outcomes, and continued controversy regarding the use of minimally invasive surgical approaches to ARM.

Minimally invasive ureteral reimplantation is an attractive and useful tool in the armamentarium for the management of complicated vesicoureteral reflux (VUR). Subureteric dextranomer/hyaluronic acid injection, laparoscopic extravesical ureteric reimplantation, and pneumovesicoscopic intravesical ureteral reimplantation with or without robotic assistance are established minimally invasive approaches for the management of VUR. The high cost and the limited availability of robotics have restricted accessibility to these approaches. Laparoscopic and/or robotic ureteral reimplantation continues to evolve and will have a significant bearing on the management of complicated VUR in infants and young children.

 Video content accompanies this article at http://www.perinatology. theclinics.com.

Transanal pull-through (TAPT) is the procedure of choice for treating Hirschsprung disease and should be performed with laparoscopic assistance using the anorectal line (ARL) to ensure optimum postoperative bowel function (POBF). The dentate line (DL) has traditionally been used as the landmark for commencing dissection during TAPT, but we prefer the ARL because the DL is too subjective and can be associated with risk for injury to delicate sensory innervation required for normal defecation in the anal transition zone. An intact anal transition zone and total excision of the posterior rectal cuff are crucial for normal defecation. Objective assessment of POBF is essential for thorough follow-up and early detection of potential late complications that may arise.

Laparoscopy is a safe and effective technique in the repair of inguinal hernias. This article describes the different laparoscopic herniorrhaphy techniques, as well as controversial topics, such as premature infants, contralateral repair, and incarcerated hernias.

PROGRAM OBJECTIVE

The goal of *Clinics in Perinatology* is to keep practicing perinatologists, neonatologists, obstetricians, practicing physicians and residents up to date with current clinical practice in perinatology by providing timely articles reviewing the state of the art in patient care.

TARGET AUDIENCE

Perinatologists, neonatologists, obstetricians, practicing physicians, residents and healthcare professionals who provide patient care utilizing findings from *Clinics in Perinatology*.

LEARNING OBJECTIVES

Upon completion of this activity, participants will be able to:

1. Review methods in minimally invasive neonatal surgery for abnormalities of the gastrointestinal system.
2. Discuss neonatal surgery for respiratory disorders.
3. Recognize developments in minimally invasive neonatal surgery techniques.

ACCREDITATION

The Elsevier Office of Continuing Medical Education (EOCME) is accredited by the Accreditation Council for Continuing Medical Education (ACCME) to provide continuing medical education for physicians.

The EOCME designates this enduring material for a maximum of 15 *AMA PRA Category 1 Credit*(s)™. Physicians should claim only the credit commensurate with the extent of their participation in the activity.

All other healthcare professionals requesting continuing education credit for this enduring material will be issued a certificate of participation.

DISCLOSURE OF CONFLICTS OF INTEREST

The EOCME assesses conflict of interest with its instructors, faculty, planners, and other individuals who are in a position to control the content of CME activities. All relevant conflicts of interest that are identified are thoroughly vetted by EOCME for fair balance, scientific objectivity, and patient care recommendations. EOCME is committed to providing its learners with CME activities that promote improvements or quality in healthcare and not a specific proprietary business or a commercial interest.

The planning committee, staff, authors and editors listed below have identified no financial relationships or relationships to products or devices they or their spouse/life partner have with commercial interest related to the content of this CME activity:

Sophia Abdulhai, MD; Sarah B. Cairo, MD, MPH; Sujit K. Chowdhary, MCh, FRCS; Matthew S. Clifton, MD, FACS, FAAP; Anjali Fortna; Alejandro V. Garcia, MD, FAAP; Ian C. Glenn, MD; Claire E. Graves, MD; Carroll M. Harmon, MD, PhD; Michael R. Harrison, MD; Kerry Holland; Caroline C.C. Hulsker, MD; Lucky Jain, MD, MBA; Hanmin Lee, MD; Leah Logan; Jeffrey Lukish, MD, FACS; Omid Madadi-Sanjani, MD; Go Miyano, MD, PhD; Jarrett Moyer, MD; Benjamin E. Padilla, MD; David H. Rothstein, MD, MS; Bethany J. Slater, MD; Biji Sreedhar, PhD; Masahiro Takeda, MD, PhD; Stefaan H.A. Tytgat, MD, PhD; Benno Ure, PhD; Subhalakshmi Vaidyanathan; David C. van der Zee, MD, PhD; Maud Y.A. van Herwaarden, MD, PhD; Lan Vu, MD; Marieke J. Witvliet, MD; Mark L. Wulkan, MD, FACS, FAAP; Atsuyuki Yamataka, MD, PhD, FAAP (Hon); Chung-Kwong Yeung, MD, PhD, FRCS, FRACS, FACS.

The planning committee, staff, authors and editors listed below have identified financial relationships or relationships to products or devices they or their spouse/life partner have with commercial interest related to the content of this CME activity:

Claus Petersen, PhD is a consultant/advisor for MedXpert.
Todd A. Ponsky, MD is a consultant/advisor for CONMED Corporation, with stock ownership in GlobalcastMD.
Steven S. Rothenberg, MD has stock ownership in JustRight Surgical, LLC.

UNAPPROVED/OFF-LABEL USE DISCLOSURE

The EOCME requires CME faculty to disclose to the participants:

1. When products or procedures being discussed are off-label, unlabelled, experimental, and/or investigational (not US Food and Drug Administration [FDA] approved); and
2. Any limitations on the information presented, such as data that are preliminary or that represent ongoing research, interim analyses, and/or unsupported opinions. Faculty may discuss information about pharmaceutical agents that is outside of FDA-approved labelling. This information is intended solely for CME and is not intended to promote off-label use of these medications. If you have any

questions, contact the medical affairs department of the manufacturer for the most recent prescribing information.

TO ENROLL

To enroll in the *Clinics in Perinatology* Continuing Medical Education program, call customer service at 1-800-654-2452 or sign up online at http://www.theclinics.com/home/cme. The CME program is available to subscribers for an additional annual fee of $235 USD.

METHOD OF PARTICIPATION

In order to claim credit, participants must complete the following:
1. Complete enrolment as indicated above.
2. Read the activity.
3. Complete the CME Test and Evaluation. Participants must achieve a score of 70% on the test. All CME Tests and Evaluations must be completed online.

CME INQUIRIES/SPECIAL NEEDS

For all CME inquiries or special needs, please contact elsevierCME@elsevier.com.

CLINICS IN PERINATOLOGY

ISSUE OF RELATED INTEREST

Pediatric Clinics of North America, April 2015 (Vol. 62, Issue 2)
The Healthy and Sick Newborn
David A. Clark, *Editor*
Available at: www.pediatric.theclinics.com

THE CLINICS ARE AVAILABLE ONLINE!
Access your subscription at:
www.theclinics.com

Erratum

An error was made in a figure in the article "Improving Neonatal Care: A Global Perspective" in the September 2017 issue of *Emergency Medicine Clinics* (44 (2017) 469-728). On Page 572, Figure 4, in the print article, included the sentence "newborn lack access" instead of "newborns lack access."

Clin Perinatol 44 (2017) xiii
https://doi.org/10.1016/j.clp.2017.09.001
0095-5108/17/© 2017 Elsevier Inc. All rights reserved.

Foreword

Minimally Invasive Surgery: Is It the Carpenter or the Tools?

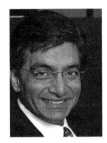

Lucky Jain, MD, MBA
Consulting Editor

The advent of motorized tools and advanced gadgets has transformed the art of wood-work and carpentry. Powerful drills and lathes have brought speed and efficiency to a historically manual trade (**Fig. 1**). As these tools become more precise and powerful, the carpenter is challenged with the need to keep up with increasingly complex oper-ator skills. Minor errors can do much harm to the finished product. The ability to touch and feel the product is often missing, forcing the operator to rely on experience and estimates. There are no randomized controlled trials to guide choices in these indus-tries. If a new tool or technique is flawed, the manufacturer issues a recall; the defective product is replaced, and life goes on.

Many parallels can be drawn between this story and the advances in minimally inva-sive surgery. Decades of steady incremental progress with traditional open surgery have created new hope for newborns and infants with congenital anomalies and other surgical needs. The introduction of minimally invasive surgeries in our NICUs in the early 1990s was received with much hope and joy.[1,2] The new technology came with a promise of less trauma, easier postoperative pain management, and better cosmetic and functional outcome. Eager to be frontrunners in the emerging field, sur-geons across the globe embraced the technology and started performing more and more complex surgeries endoscopically.[2] Even seemingly inaccessible areas such as pediatric neurosurgery have seen major intraoperative technological advances that include the microscope, which has allowed precise surgery under magnification and improved lighting, and the endoscope, which has improved the treatment of hy-drocephalus and allowed biopsy and complete resection of intraventricular, pituitary, and pineal region tumors through a minimally invasive approach.[3] Rigorous random-ized trials comparing these new approaches to traditional open surgeries were not al-ways available, and surgeons used the "feasibility" doctrine to drive change with the broad assumption that "if it can be done endoscopically, it will likely be better."[4] Little

Clin Perinatol 44 (2017) xv–xvii
https://doi.org/10.1016/j.clp.2017.09.003
0095-5108/17/© 2017 Published by Elsevier Inc.

perinatology.theclinics.com

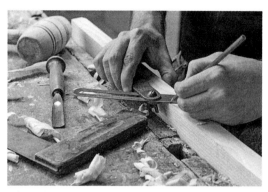

Fig. 1. Carpenter with tools.

attention was paid to newer centers with low volumes and less experienced operators, and it was hard to monitor their outcomes. Neonatologists who historically have been sticklers about randomized trials were surprisingly eager to play along, and parents, often unaware of these issues, went with the lure of the new technology and better cosmetic outcomes.

Initial reports of outcomes were limited to case reports and small series. Reports of outcomes using large databases and registries are beginning to make their way into the literature and present a mixed picture. For most applications, minimally invasive surgery appears to have improved outcomes. A recent review of congenital thoracic anomalies shows easier postoperative care and shorter length of stay.[5] Other studies however have shown higher rates of recurrence after laparoscopic surgery.[6] What is not factored in these outcomes is the lack of a credible denominator. True representative data would need to be derived from all participating centers, big and small, not just high-volume leaders reporting outcomes.

Robotic surgery has now emerged as a new frontier, presenting the same challenges and opportunities as minimally invasive surgery did decades ago.[7] While robotic surgery offers considerable technical advantages over conventional laparoscopy and is associated with only a modest learning curve, the improvement in clinical outcomes is marginal and there are several disadvantages. There are increased setup and operating times, need to accommodate and maintain large sophisticated equipment, and requirement for additional training.

Overall, it is comforting to know that unlike early adopters of minimally invasive surgery who struggled between the two approaches, a large majority of newly minted surgeons are appropriately trained in both techniques and can individualize choices to patients and conditions. Like any new technique, endoscopic surgery continues to evolve and improve. Newer applications in complex conditions such as cardiac valve repair and congenital diaphragmatic hernias reflect increasing operator comfort and promise of better outcomes.

I am very fortunate to have worked with two leaders in this field, Drs Wulkan and Lee, who have also taken on the onus of putting together this issue of *Clinics in Perinatology* for you. Together, they have done a phenomenal job in putting together a series of articles on minimally invasive surgery. As always, I am grateful to editorial team at Elsevier, led by Kerry Holland and Casey Potter, for bringing this important publication to you.

Lucky Jain, MD, MBA
Department of Pediatrics
Emory University School of Medicine
Children's Healthcare of Atlanta
2015 Uppergate Drive
Atlanta, GA 30322, USA

E-mail address:
ljain@emory.edu

REFERENCES

1. Davenport M, Rothenberg SS, Crabbe DC, et al. The great debate: open or thoracoscopic repair for oesophageal atresia or diaphragmatic hernia. J Pediatr Surg 2015;50(2):240–6.
2. Lacher M, Kuebler JF, Dingemann J, et al. Minimal invasive surgery in the newborn: current status and evidence. Semin Pediatr Surg 2014;23(5):249–56.
3. Zebian B, Vergani F, Lavrador JP, et al. Recent technological advances in pediatric brain tumor surgery. CNS Oncol 2017;6(1):71–82.
4. Schwartz JA. Innovation in pediatric surgery: the surgical innovation continuum and the ethical model. J Pediatr Surg 2014;49:639–45.
5. Adams S, Jobson M, Sangnawakij P, et al. Does thoracoscopy have advantages over open surgery for asymptomatic congenital lung malformations? An analysis of 1626 resections. J Pediatr Surg 2017;52(2):247–51.
6. Terui K, Nagata K, Ito M, et al. Surgical approaches for neonatal congenital diaphragmatic hernia: a systematic review and meta-analysis. Pediatr Surg Int 2015;31(10):891–7.
7. Nicklin J. The future of robotic-assisted laparoscopic gynaecologic surgery in Australia—a time and a place for everything. Aust N Z J Obstet Gynaecol 2017. https://doi.org/10.1111/ajo.12688.

Preface

Minimally Invasive Neonatal Surgery

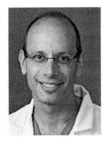 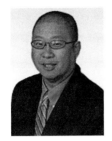

Mark L. Wulkan, MD   Hanmin Lee, MD
Editors

This issue of *Clinics in Perinatology* is focused on minimally invasive surgical techniques in the newborn patient. In the 1990s, minimally invasive surgery was developed for infants and children. As technology has improved, we are now able to perform complex *minimally invasive* operations on our smallest, most vulnerable patients. High-definition video and miniature instrumentation allow us to routinely perform congenital diaphragmatic hernia repair, correction of esophageal atresia, pull-through for imperforate anus, and other procedures as outlined in this issue. We are grateful for the experts from around the world who have agreed to contribute to this issue. Our goal is for perinatologists, neonatologists, pediatricians, and pediatric surgeons to understand what is now possible. Our patients experience less pain, shorter ventilator days, and potentially shorter hospital stays due to their expertise.

Mark L. Wulkan, MD
Pediatric Surgery
Emory Univeristy School of Medicine
Children's Healthcare of Atlanta
1405 Clifton Road
Atlanta, GA 30322, USA

Hanmin Lee, MD
Pediatric Surgery
University of California–San Francisco
550 16th Street, 5th Floor
UCSF Box 0570
San Francisco, CA 94143, USA

E-mail addresses:
mwulkan@emory.edu (M.L. Wulkan)
hanmin.lee@ucsf.edu (H. Lee)

Clin Perinatol 44 (2017) xix
https://doi.org/10.1016/j.clp.2017.09.002
0095-5108/17/© 2017 Published by Elsevier Inc.

Minimally Invasive Fetal Surgery

Claire E. Graves, MD[a], Michael R. Harrison, MD[b], Benjamin E. Padilla, MD[c],*

KEYWORDS

- Fetal surgery • Fetal therapy • Fetal diagnosis • Prenatal diagnosis
- Fetoscopic surgery • Fetoscopy

KEY POINTS

- The goal of minimally invasive fetal treatments is to decrease maternal risk and premature rupture of membranes.
- Real-time ultrasound imaging is crucial to the implementation and success of minimally invasive fetal procedures.
- Multidisciplinary fetal procedural teams, including a fetal surgeon, ultrasonographer, perinatologist, and anesthesiologist, are critical to the delivery of quality care.

INTRODUCTION: NATURE OF THE PROBLEM
History and General Principles

In the past 50 years, fetal therapy has progressed from mere concept to an accepted and viable treatment modality. A better understanding of embryology and fetal development, coupled with the advent of high-resolution noninvasive fetal imaging, led to a fundamental shift in thinking of the fetus itself as a patient.[1] With earlier and more accurate diagnosis of many congenital defects, the window of opportunity for intervention widened. Throughout the second half of the 20th century, physician and surgeon scientists took a rigorous scientific approach in tackling the problem of fetal surgery: identifying the clinical need, studying the natural history of diseases in the human fetus, understanding the pathophysiology and proposed treatments in the laboratory, and safely implementing fetal interventions in humans. Through these efforts, fetal therapy has improved survival and decreased morbidity for many devastating congenital defects, while minimizing risk to the mother. Technical advances, coupled with

Disclosure Statement: The authors have nothing to disclose.
^a Department of Surgery, University of California, San Francisco, 550 16th Street 5th Floor UCSF Mail Stop 0570, San Francisco, CA 94158-2549, USA; ^b University of California, San Francisco, 550 16th Street 5th Floor UCSF Mail Stop 0570, San Francisco, CA 94158-2549, USA; ^c Division of Pediatric Surgery, Department of Surgery, University of California, San Francisco, 550 16th Street 5th Floor UCSF Mail Stop 0570, San Francisco, CA 94158-2549, USA
* Corresponding author.
E-mail address: Benjamin.Padilla@ucsf.edu

Clin Perinatol 44 (2017) 729–751
http://dx.doi.org/10.1016/j.clp.2017.08.001   **perinatology.theclinics.com**
0095-5108/17/© 2017 Elsevier Inc. All rights reserved.

ongoing efforts to make fetal procedures safer for the mother, have led to ongoing innovation in the field, including the development of minimally invasive therapies and procedures.

Although many minimally invasive fetal operations are simply adaptations of the open operation, others were developed specifically for minimally invasive techniques. Indeed, some can only be performed in this way. The first modern fetal intervention was needle based. In 1963, Liley performed the first fetal transfusion by inserting a 16-G Touhy needle into the fetal peritoneal space.[2] In this era before modern ultrasound imaging, Liley localized the fetal abdomen by injecting contrast into the amniotic cavity and allowing it to be swallowed by the fetus to opacify the fetal bowel. Given the success of this needle-based technique, enthusiasm for existing open transfusion procedures waned.[3] In the 1970s, direct visualization of the fetus with endoscopy was first introduced for diagnostic purposes, such as to obtain fetal blood or biopsy tissue, but therapeutic use was limited because of its invasiveness and the technical skill required.[4] Fetoscopic diagnosis became essentially obsolete when ultrasound examination became more widespread, shifting instead to percutaneous needle-based techniques under ultrasound guidance. It was not until the early 1990s, when smaller cameras and endoscopes coupled with the increasing popularity of laparoscopic surgery, led to a resurgence of interest in fetoscopic and minimal access procedures.[4–7] **Box 1** highlights some milestones in the development of minimally invasive fetal procedures. Some of the early challenges in the development of these techniques have been summarized elsewhere.[8]

Ethical Considerations

Fetal intervention raises unique ethical issues surrounding maternal autonomy and decision making. Although the goal of fetal intervention is to cure or better the health of the fetus, any intervention, whether surgical or pharmacologic, necessarily affects the pregnant mother. The pregnant woman gains nothing in terms of personal health benefits, and the unborn child gets all potential benefit. Protecting the pregnant woman and mitigating risk is the greatest responsibility of fetal therapy teams. Therefore, explicit informed consent is required for all fetal interventions, and must be obtained with a comprehensive discussion of her unique risks. Moreover, women must also be informed of, and provided access to, alternatives to intervention, including postnatal therapy, palliative care, or pregnancy termination in a nondirective manner.[9,10]

Innovation in fetal therapy, including the development of minimally invasive procedures, is necessary to continue to expand the benefits of fetal treatment and reduce risks to pregnant women. However, formal clinical research in this population is often

Box 1	
Milestones in the development of minimally invasive fetal surgery	
Milestone	**Year**
First fetal transfusion	1963
First fetal vesicoamniotic shunt placement	1982
First open fetal surgery	1982
First fetal thoracoamniotic shunt placement	1987
First laser ablation for twin–twin transfusion syndrome	1990
First fetoscopic repair of myelomeningocele	1997
First "Fetendo" tracheal clipping for congenital diaphragmatic hernia	1997
First fetoscopic release of amniotic band	1997
First fetoscopic balloon tracheal occlusion for congenital diaphragmatic hernia	2001

difficult, owing to the lack of appropriate animal models in some diseases, as well as small patient numbers. Therefore, fetal innovation benefits from collaboration between and among disciplines as well as between multiple centers. To guide practitioners in responsible innovation, the North American Fetal Therapy Network has developed guidelines regarding medical innovation in maternal–fetal therapy.[11]

SURGICAL TECHNIQUES AND PROCEDURES
Surgical Team

In fetal surgery, in which there are complex diseases and multiple patients, careful planning and open communication before, during, and after surgery between the members of the multidisciplinary care team are essential. The disciplines that may be involved include pediatric surgery, obstetrics, pediatric anesthesia, obstetric anesthesia, cardiology, radiology, otolaryngology, neonatology, neonatal nursing, and operative room nursing.[12] At our institution, regular, weekly multidisciplinary meetings are held to discuss upcoming patients and come to consensus on treatment plans.

During most minimally invasive procedures, ultrasound imaging is used to provide guidance to the proceduralist (usually a pediatric surgeon and/or obstetrician) and to monitor the fetus during surgery. These practitioners actively communicate with the anesthesia team, as well as nursing and scrub staff, throughout the procedure. Owing to the specialized equipment required, an active and knowledgeable technical support staff is essential.

Surgical Approach

Minimally invasive fetal surgery is broadly divided into 2 categories: (1) needle based and (2) fetoscopic. For both, the mother is usually positioned supine with the right side angled up or elevated with a bump to minimize compression of the inferior vena cava. Intraoperative, real-time ultrasound imaging is critical to both types of procedures. Upon initial access, it is used to identify a safe entry point on the uterus, free of large vessels and placental attachments. To minimize the risk of bleeding, placental abruption, and fetal morbidity, traversing the placenta is avoided if at all possible. Ultrasound imaging is also important for determining the location and position of the fetus and assessing its well-being throughout the operation by monitoring fetal heart function and umbilical artery blood flow.

Minimally invasive fetal operations are performed through a small skin incision on the mother's abdomen. The location of the incision is based on the position of the placenta, as well as the intrauterine target. The needles used to access the fetus are approximately 1 to 2 mm in diameter, as small as possible to minimize maternal morbidity. In cases of anterior placenta, curved instruments may be used to access target structures.[13] Through needle-based fetal access, fluid associated with ascites, pleural effusions, cystic structures, or the bladder can be aspirated or drained with a shunt into the amniotic space. In addition, needle-based access is used in fetal cardiac valvuloplasty and ablative procedures, such as radiofrequency ablation (RFA) in the management of complications of twin gestation.

Fetoscopic procedures are usually performed via a single 2.3- to 4.0-mm (7- to 12-Fr) port that accommodates 1.2- to 3-mm endoscopes, with or without a working channel (**Fig. 1**).[8] When only a single access port is used, a small skin incision is made on the mother's abdomen to access the uterus. When multiple ports are required, multiple small incisions may be made, or the uterus may be visualized through a larger laparotomy before port insertion. The scope can be inserted directly into the amniotic cavity using a sharp trocar within the sheath of the fetoscope itself, or a cannula

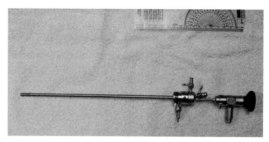

Fig. 1. Fetoscopic procedures are performed using 1.2- to 3.0-mm endoscopes. Pictured is a 3 mm 0° endoscope, adjustable length, with a 1-mm working channel.

can first be inserted to create a working port, either with a trocar or via Seldinger technique.[14] Again, ultrasound imaging is essential for safe uterine access and is an adjunct to the fetoscope for visualizing the fetus. If the amniotic fluid is not clear enough to allow for a good image via a small endoscope, amnio-exchange with warmed crystalloid solution may improve visualization. The fetoscopic technique is currently used when direct visualization is required in addition to ultrasonography, for example, in the treatment of twin–twin transfusion syndrome (TTTS), posterior urethral valves (PUV), constricting amniotic bands, and tracheal balloon occlusion for congenital diaphragmatic hernia (CDH).

Anesthetic Considerations

Anesthesia during fetal procedures is based on an understanding of both maternal and fetal physiology.[12] Minimally invasive fetal procedures require varying degrees of maternal analgesia and anesthesia, as well as fetal analgesia and/or immobility, depending on procedure complexity and the instrumentation required.

Typically, needle-based and single port fetoscopic procedures are well-tolerated by the mother under local anesthesia. For complex procedures requiring multiple ports or when backup Caesarian section could be necessary, regional anesthesia such as epidural or combined spinal epidural anesthesia may be used.[15,16] The fetus does not receive any anesthesia or analgesia from maternal local or regional techniques. Therefore, additional fetal anesthesia is usually required for endoscopic procedures performed directly on the fetus. Fetal anesthesia is typically administered intramuscularly and consists of opiates and nondepolarizing muscle relaxants.[12,15] Atropine is often given simultaneously to prevent fetal bradycardia.[17] For procedures on the placenta or cord, which do not have direct contact with the fetus, the risks of fetal anesthesia likely outweigh the benefits.

Complications

The complications of minimally invasive fetal surgery are similar to those of open fetal surgery, including bleeding, amniotic fluid leak, chorioamnionic separation, chorioamnionitis, premature rupture of membranes (PROM)/preterm prelabor rupture of membranes (PPROM), preterm birth, and fetal demise. PROM/PPROM is the most common complication of minimally invasive fetal surgery, with potentially significant morbidity, including oligohydramnios, chorioamnionitis, and preterm delivery. However, accurate analysis of the frequency of PROM and PPROM in these procedures is made difficult by the variations in both the assessment of the complication as well as reporting methods.[18] In TTTS, the rate of PROM is estimated at approximately 26% to 40%.[14,18,19] Complications of other procedures are discussed further elsewhere in this article.

Factors affecting the morbidity of minimally invasive fetal procedures include the number of ports used and the diameter of the instruments. A systematic review of 1376 minimally invasive fetal procedures for TTTS, lower urinary tract obstruction (LUTO), and twin reversed arterial perfusion (TRAP) sequence identified maximum diameter of the instrument and maximum number of ports as predictors of iatrogenic PPROM.[18] Maximum instrument diameter also significantly decreased gestational age at birth. Though there was initially great enthusiasm that multiport fetoscopic surgery, with smaller uterine incisions, would decrease morbidity, multiport fetoscopic surgery has thus far proven disappointing. In the largest experience with multiport fetoscopic surgery, myelomeningocele (MMC) repair, this technique has yet to decrease complications when compared with open surgery.[20–23]

Although fetal surgery has not been demonstrated to have an adverse effect on future fertility,[24] open fetal surgery requires planned Caesarian delivery before labor for the affected fetus and future pregnancies to prevent dehiscence at the fetal surgery hysterotomy scar. This factor does increase the risk of delivery complications and is a critical aspect of maternal counseling.[25] Importantly, minimally invasive fetal surgery does not preclude vaginal delivery. Although the long-term follow-up of subsequent pregnancies after these procedures is lacking, avoiding the complications of repeat Caesarian section is considered a significant advantage of minimally invasive procedures.

SPECIFIC CONDITIONS AND MINIMALLY INVASIVE PROCEDURES
Twin Gestations

Twin–twin transfusion syndrome
TTTS is a severe complication of monochorionic pregnancies that arises from an imbalance of flow through intertwin placental vascular anastomoses. Clinical effects, generally not seen until the second trimester, are related to a discrepancy in the intravascular volume. The donor twin develops hypovolemia, leading to oliguria and oligohydramnios from reduced renal perfusion, and the recipient twin suffers the consequences of hypervolemia, including polyuria and polyhydramnios.[26] Both twins are at risk for significant morbidity: the donor from hypoxic–ischemic injuries and growth restriction, and the recipient from cardiac decompensation and hydrops. In addition, these babies frequently suffer from long-term neurodevelopmental complications.[27] Disease severity is staged using clinical and ultrasonographic criteria developed by Quintero and colleagues[28] (**Table 1**). If left untreated, severe TTTS is lethal, with perinatal mortality rates of up to 80% to 90%.[26,29,30]

Table 1	
Staging of twin–twin transfusion syndrome	
Stage	**Ultrasound/Doppler Findings**
I	Polyhydramnios and oligohydramnios
II	Stage I plus donor bladder not visualized
III	Stage II plus critically abnormal Doppler (umbilical artery absent or reversed end-diastolic velocity, ductus venosus reversed flow, pulsatile umbilical venous flow)
IV	Stage III plus hydrops
V	Fetal demise

Adapted from Quintero RA, Morales WJ, Allen MH, et al. Staging of twin-twin transfusion syndrome. J Perinatol 1999;19:550–5.

Initial interventions for TTTS focused on removing the excess amniotic fluid surrounding the recipient twin, with the goals of preventing preterm delivery secondary to polyhydramnios and improving fetal circulation by decreasing pressure on the chorionic plate.[30,31] In 1990, an alternative procedure was proposed that used a fetoscopic laser to coagulate the superficial blood vessels that cross the separating membrane of the placenta, separating the 2 fetal circulations and destroying the intertwin vessels that cause discordant twin–twin transfusion.[32] Currently, placental laser ablation is the preferred treatment of TTTS between 16 and 26 weeks of gestation. The procedure is performed through a single uterine access site using a fetoscope and thin laser fiber (**Fig. 2**).

The superiority of laser ablation compared with amnioreduction was first demonstrated in 2004, when a multicenter, randomized, controlled trial by the Eurofoetus Consortium compared selective laser ablation with serial amnioreduction in severe TTTS between 16 and 26 weeks of gestation.[29] Patients treated with laser ablation had a significantly higher survival rate of at least 1 twin to 6 months of age (76% vs 51%; P = .002). Moreover, twins treated with laser ablation were more likely to be free of neurologic complications at 6 months of age (52% vs 31%; P = .003). These data were pooled in a 2014 Cochrane review with a 2007 multicenter, randomized, controlled trial in the United States, sponsored by the National Institute of Child Health and Human Development.[33] This review found no difference in overall death between the laser ablation and amnioreduction groups (relative risk [RR], 0.87; 95% CI, 0.55–1.38), but did report a higher percentage of babies alive at 6 years of age without neurologic abnormality in the laser group (RR, 1.57; 95% CI, 1.05–2.34). The authors of the Cochrane review concluded that endoscopic laser coagulation of anastomotic vessels should continue to be considered in the treatment of all stages of TTTS to

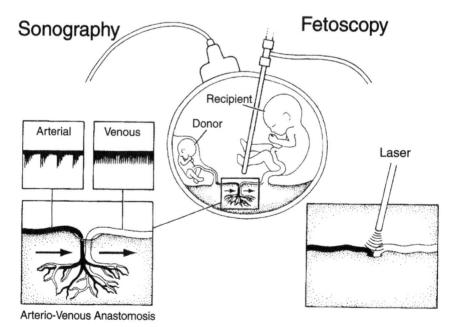

Fig. 2. Diagram of fetoscopic laser ablation for twin–twin transfusion syndrome. Under ultrasound guidance, a fetoscope is placed into the amniotic space. Using both ultrasound guidance and fetoscopic visualization, intertwin vessels are destroyed with laser ablation.

improve neurodevelopmental outcomes.[30] Although some debate exists over whether the benefit outweighs the risks of intervention in stage I TTTS, a recent multicenter, retrospective review demonstrated improved outcomes with prenatal intervention (amnioreduction or laser) over observation.[34]

Selective fetal reduction

In addition to TTTS, monochorionic twin pregnancies are susceptible to a variety of other serious complications, including selective intrauterine growth restriction, structural anomalies, twin anemia polycythemia sequence, and TRAP sequence, or acardiac twinning.[35] In some complicated monochorionic pregnancies at high risk of hemodynamic compromise or intrauterine fetal death, elective fetal reduction is recommended to prevent neurologic injury or demise of the cotwin.[36,37] Because of risk of transmission between twins, fetal intracardiac potassium chloride injection is contraindicated in these pregnancies, and selective termination must be performed with interruption of blood flow to the fetus. Methods used to achieve this have included ligation of the umbilical cord, fetoscopic laser coagulation, ultrasound-guided bipolar cord coagulation, and RFA (**Fig. 3**).[38]

   The most convincing evidence for benefit of selective reduction in complicated twin pregnancies has been demonstrated for TRAP sequence. In TRAP sequence, 1 twin has an absent or rudimentary heart, as well as absence of other vital structures, including the head, making it incompatible with life. This twin has no placental share, and it receives its blood supply through direct vascular connections from the normal or "pump" twin. Left untreated, the normal twin develops high-output cardiac failure, resulting in greater than 50% mortality.[39] By stopping flow to the acardiac twin, the normal twin is protected. In the largest series to date, a 2013 review of the North American Fetal Therapy Network registry data from 12 fetal centers identified 98 patients who underwent percutaneous RFA of an acardiac twin.[39] In this series, the overall survival of the pump twin to 30 days was 80%.

Lower Urinary Tract Obstruction

Congenital LUTO is most often caused by PUV, urethral atresia, or the prune belly syndrome.[40] The condition is usually diagnosed on routine prenatal screening ultrasound examination, typically performed at 20 weeks' gestation. Hallmarks of diagnosis include a dilated bladder with thickened bladder wall, as well as dilation of the

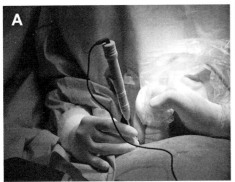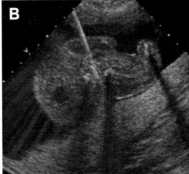

Fig. 3. Radiofrequency ablation (RFA) of the cord of an anomalous twin in a monochorionic pregnancy. (*A*) External view of maternal abdomen with ultrasound and RFA probes. (*B*) Sonographic view of probe aimed at umbilicus of target fetus.

posterior urethra—the "keyhole sign."[41] When associated with early oligohydramnios, consequent pulmonary hypoplasia can lead to perinatal mortality of up to 50%,[42] and children who survive are at high risk for chronic kidney disease or end-stage renal disease.[43]

The basis of fetal intervention on LUTO is that the relief of urinary obstruction and resultant increase in amniotic fluid promotes lung development and maturity.[44] Moreover, animal models of LUTO indicate that renal damage caused by outflow obstruction is greater the earlier in gestation it occurs and the longer it is sustained.[45,46] The first fetal interventions for congenital LUTO were developed in the fetal lamb and primate models, and then translated to human treatment at the University of California San Francisco in the early 1980s.[44,47–49] These early interventions initially involved open fetal procedures with cutaneous ureterostomies, as well as minimally invasive approaches such as ultrasound-guided aspiration of fetal urine through needles or catheters and internal drainage through indwelling shunts.

Currently, 2 main techniques are used in specialized centers. In the first, vesicoamniotic shunting (VAS), a double pigtail stent is placed percutaneously under ultrasound guidance, usually in conjunction with amnioinfusion (**Fig. 4**). The second technique is fetal cystoscopy, in which a fetoscope is placed through a trocar within the fetal bladder, to diagnose the source of obstruction and to ablate PUV. Various methods have been used to ablate the valve, including guide wires, hydroablation, and laser ablation.[50]

Table 2 summarizes recent studies on minimally invasive therapy for LUTO. Initial reports of VAS consisted of small case series using a variety of surgical techniques and different criteria for fetal selection. A metaanalysis of these early studies through 2002, which included a total of 342 fetuses, suggested that bladder drainage improved perinatal survival (odds ratio, 2.5; $P = .03$), most markedly in fetuses with poor prognoses.[51] However, complications of shunting included failure of placement, catheter occlusion, dislocation, and fistula. To more rigorously evaluate the effect of in utero VAS, and gather data on long-term outcomes in these infants, a multinational, randomized, controlled trial, "Percutaneous vesicoamniotic shunting versus conservative management for fetal Lower Urinary Tract Obstruction" (PLUTO), was performed in the United Kingdom, Ireland, and the Netherlands from 2006 to 2012.[52] Although planned enrollment was 150, the study closed early with only 31 participants (16 assigned to VAS, 15 to conservative management) because of recruitment

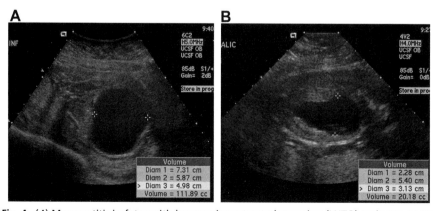

Fig. 4. (*A*) Megacystitis in fetus with lower urinary tract obstruction (LUTO) owing to posterior urethral valves (PUV). (*B*) Decompressed bladder 2 days after fetoscopic valve ablation.

Table 2
Selected reports of minimally invasive fetal intervention for lower urinary tract obstruction

Authors	Year	Design	N	Outcomes
Ruano et al,[41] 2010	2010	Retrospective single institution: cystoscopy vs expectant management	23	Improved survival (62.5%) vs (11.1%) with prenatal cystoscopy; normal postnatal renal function in 62.5% after cystoscopy vs 11.1% in control
Morris et al,[52] 2013	2013	Prospective randomized: VAS vs observation	31	Trend toward improved survival with VAS (RR, 1.88); poor long-term outcomes; 2/31 (6.4%) with normal renal function at 2 y (29% of survivors)
Ruano et al,[53] 2015	2015	Retrospective multicenter: cystoscopy vs VAS vs observation	111	Significantly improved survival with fetal intervention cystoscopy (adjusted RR, 1.86) and VAS (adjusted RR, 1.73) vs observation; trend toward improved renal function with cystoscopy, but not with VAS
Sananes et al,[54] 2016	2016	Retrospective multicenter cohort: cystoscopy	50	Overall survival at 1 y (37.5%). In cohort with PUV ablation, 1-y survival (56.7%), normal renal function at 2 y: 25.0% of original cohort, 75.0% of survivors

Abbreviations: PUV, posterior urethral valves; RR, relative risk; VAS, vesicoamniotic shunting.

difficulties. Preterm labor, number of live births, or neonatal requirement of ventilation did not differ significantly between the 2 groups. Survival to 28 days was better in the VAS group (intention-to-treat RR, 1.88 [P = .27]; as-treated RR, 3.20 [P = .03]), but long-term clinical outcomes were poor in both groups, with only 2 infants having normal renal function at 1 and 2 years (both in the VAS group). The authors suggest that irreversible damage to the renal parenchyma may take place before the time of diagnosis.

Although more invasive than VAS, fetal cystoscopy has the advantage of confirming the diagnosis of PUV, and thus more accurately selecting patients who will benefit from valve ablation. In a recent multicenter retrospective cohort study of 50 fetal cystoscopies for LUTO, 30 fetuses were found to have PUV and were treated with pulsed Nd:YAG laser ablation; the 20 remaining fetuses were diagnosed with urethral atresia (n = 13), urethral stenosis (n = 5), or trisomy 18 (n = 2) and were not treated.[54] Of the 48 patients with normal karyotype, mean gestational age at delivery was 32.4 weeks, and overall survival to 2 years was 34.8%. For patients with PUV treated with laser ablation, survival to 2 years was 53.6%, although 6 of the 30 (20%) had recurrence of LUTO, and an additional fetal procedure was performed in 3 patients (10%). Ten of the 17 survivors underwent additional postnatal ablation of PUV. At 2 years of age, 12 of the 16 infants (75%) with PUV had normal renal function, which is far more promising than the 29% reported in the PLUTO trial with VAS.

Evidence to date suggests that, in selected cases of LUTO, minimally invasive fetal therapy may improve survival compared with expectant management. However, reports of long-term renal function have been disappointing. The improved renal function with cystoscopy and valve ablation in the cohorts of patients with confirmed PUV[53,54] have led some practitioners to propose cystoscopy as a first-line intervention for diagnosis as well as valve ablation when PUV is confirmed. Patients with urethral stenosis, who are not candidates for ablation, could be considered for VAS.

Minimally Invasive Repair of Myelomeningocele

MMC, or spina bifida, is characterized by incomplete closure of the neural tube and exposure of the spinal canal elements. MMC can occur anywhere along the spine, but most commonly affects the lumbar or cervical vertebral levels. Complications include neurologic deficits with motor and somatosensory abnormalities. In addition, injury to the autonomic nervous system can impede bowel and bladder function. Finally, nearly all patients with MMC develop the Arnold-Chiari II malformation of the hindbrain, which results in noncommunicating hydrocephalus and requires ventriculo-peritoneal shunting. Although MMC has low mortality in the perinatal period, the long-term morbidity from neurologic abnormalities is severe, and up to 30% of patients die before reaching adulthood.[55]

Fetal intervention in MMC is based on the "2-hit" hypothesis of the neurologic injury, where the first hit is the neural tube defect itself, and the second hit is trauma to the exposed neural elements while the fetus is in utero.[56,57] Fetal surgery aims to intervene before secondary damage can occur to the exposed structures. Animal models of fetal MMC, primarily in sheep, proved this hypothesis and showed that in utero repair of the MMC improved distal neurologic function and reversed the Arnold-Chiari II malformation.[58–60]

MMC was the first nonlethal anomaly to be treated with fetal surgery.[55,61] The first minimally invasive in utero coverage of MMC was performed in 1997, with endoscopic placement of a maternal split-thickness skin graft over the fetal neural placode.[62] These early fetoscopic repairs were complicated by a high rate of fetal death (50%),[63] and efforts shifted to refining an open technique via hysterotomy. These open fetal procedures were promising, demonstrating decreased hindbrain herniation and improved neurologic function.[64,65] To rigorously assess the benefit of fetal surgery on MMC, the National Institutes of Health sponsored a multicenter randomized trial, Management of Myelomeningocele Study (MOMS), comparing fetal MMC repair at 19 to 26 weeks gestation with conventional postnatal repair.[66] The study closed early because of the superiority of fetal surgery. Fetal MMC repair reduced the need for ven-triculoperitoneal shunting for hydrocephalus at 1 year (fetal group, 40% vs postnatal group, 82%; $P<.001$) and improved motor function, including the ability to walk at 30 months of age (fetal group, 42% vs postnatal group, 21%; $P<.01$). Fetuses treated prenatally were born at an average gestational age of 34.1 weeks of gestation and 13% were born before 30 weeks of gestation.

Although the MOMS trial decisively demonstrated the value of in utero repair of MMC, the morbidity of the disease was still substantial, with 40% of patients in the prenatal group requiring shunts. Moreover, maternal complications in the prenatal sur-gery group included spontaneous membrane rupture (46%), chorioamniotic mem-brane separation (26%), and placental abruption (6%). Therefore, techniques to improve prenatal repair, including fetoscopic techniques, continue to be investigated.

Two fetoscopic techniques have been recently reported. The first uses three or four 5-mm trocars, placed in the amniotic cavity via Seldinger technique under ultra-sound guidance.[20] Partial amniotic carbon dioxide insufflation is performed after removal of a portion of the amniotic fluid to provide visibility throughout the proced-ure. The malformation is dissected with a needle electrode, and the placode is manu-ally dissected free from surrounding tissues with microscissors and micrograsper. Depending on the anatomy of the lesion, the neural tissue is covered with 1 or more Teflon and collagen patches. The results of a review of 51 cases with this technique (some outcomes reported in expanded series of 71 cases) are summarized in **Table 3** and compared with results from the open fetal surgery cohort in the MOMS trial. In the case series, 2 early infant deaths were reported from severe brainstem dysfunction owing to Chiari II malformation, which is not seen after open fetal surgery.[67] Additionally, 28% of patients required postnatal recoverage procedures. The rate of amniotic fluid leakage (PROM) after the procedure was 84%, at a mean gestational age of 29.7 weeks, indicating that smaller access sites fail to lessen this complication.

A second technique uses smaller access sites, with two 11-Fr vascular introducers and a third 14-Fr or 16-Fr vascular introducer (or a 5-mm laparoscopic trocar).[23] After partial CO_2 insufflation, the neural placode is released and surrounding skin undermined using 3-mm laparoscopic instruments and a 2.7- to 4.0-mm endoscope. The placode is covered with a biocelluose patch (not sutured in place), and the skin is closed with a 2-0 nonabsorbable monofilament suture. A skin substitute is used for 2-layer closure in larger defects. In a phase I human trial of 10 fetal repairs with this technique, 2 procedures were aborted owing to trocar displacement, with one of these cases resulting in intrauterine death 3 days after surgery owing to severe maternal preeclampsia. Mean gestational age at delivery in the remaining cases was 32.4 weeks, with PROM occurring in all cases at a mean gestational age of 30.2 weeks. One neonatal death occurred from sepsis owing to necrotizing enterocolitis. Two cases underwent early postnatal neurosurgical repair, and 3 cases met the criteria for ventriculoperitoneal shunting within 1 year.

Open fetal MMC repair has been rigorously studied and the benefits to the fetus have been proven. Minimally invasive fetoscopic repair is technically difficult, carries high rates of membrane separation and PROM, and the benefits of this technique to

Table 3
Comparison of outcomes of minimally invasive MMC repair and open fetal surgery

Outcome	MOMS Trial, Prenatal Surgery cohort[66] (n = 78), n (%)	Case Series Review by Kohl et al[20–22] (n = 51),[a] n (%)
Aborted procedure	0	1 (2)
Chorioamniotic membrane separation	20 (26)	1 (2)
Maternal chorioamnionitis	2 (3)	4 (8)
Spontaneous membrane rupture/amniotic fluid leakage	26 (46)	43 (84)
Placental abruption	5 (6)	0
Mean gestational age at delivery (wk ± SD)	34.1 ± 3.1	33.0 ± 2.8
Gestational age at birth of <30 wk	10 (13)	9 (13)[a]
Gestational age at birth of >35 wk	42 (54)	17 (23)[a]
Perinatal deaths	2 (3)	4 (8)
Death within first year of life	2 (3)	5 (7)[a]
Postnatal re-coverage required	N/A	20 (28)[a]
Shunt required within first year of life	Criteria met: 51 (65) Shunt placed: 31 (40)	32 (45)[a]
Chiari decompression surgery	1 (1)	3 (4)[a]

Abbreviations: MMC, myelomeningocele; MOMS, Management of Myelomeningocele Study; N/A, not applicable.
[a] Outcomes reported in expanded series; n = 71.

the unborn child have not been rigorously substantiated. In light of these facts, minimally invasive MMC repair should be considered experimental until further validated.

Congenital Diaphragmatic Hernia

CDH occurs in approximately 1 in 2500 live births and consists of a defect in the fetal diaphragm, leading to herniation of abdominal viscera into the thoracic cavity.[68] Abnormal development of the lungs and pulmonary vasculature results in pulmonary hypoplasia and pulmonary hypertension, which in turn can result in persistent fetal circulation and respiratory failure. Despite advances in neonatal care, the mortality of infants with isolated CDH remains 20% to 30%.[69,70] Sonographic indicators of poor prognosis include a low lung-to-head ratio and the presence of liver herniation into the thoracic cavity, and fetal MRI has been used to determine total lung volume in these fetuses.[70]

The goal of fetal intervention in CDH is to counteract the pulmonary effects of the anomaly and promote lung growth in utero. Open fetal repair of CDH was technically feasible, but surgery in fetuses with poor prognosis liver herniation was fraught with high mortality despite treatment, and fetuses with better prognosis (no liver herniation) were just as effectively managed with postnatal repair.[71,72] These disappointing results prompted new approaches to reverse lung hypoplasia. Based on the observation that fetuses with congenital high airway obstruction or laryngeal atresia are born with hyperplastic lungs,[73] it was hypothesized that tracheal occlusion in utero would promote lung growth in fetuses with CDH (**Fig. 5**). This hypothesis was tested extensively in the fetal lamb model of CDH using various methods of tracheal occlusion, including suture ligation,[74,75] foam-cuffed endotracheal tubes, and expandable foam inserts.[76] Tracheal occlusion in the fetal lamb model of CDH increased lung volume, decreased herniation of abdominal viscera, and improved postnatal lung function.[74,75] The effect of in utero tracheal occlusion on lung growth was later corroborated in a rat model of CDH.[77,78]

In utero tracheal occlusion was first performed in humans in 1996 via maternal laparotomy and open hysterotomy.[79] However, the large hysterotomy required for adequate fetal exposure led to a high rate of preterm labor. Therefore, fetal

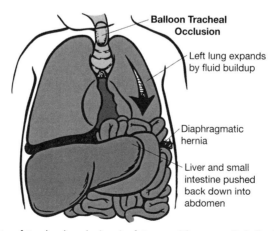

Fig. 5. The effects of tracheal occlusion in fetuses with congenital diaphragmatic hernia (CDH). Occluding the trachea of fetuses with CDH increases lung volume, decreases herniation of abdominal viscera, and improves postnatal lung function.

surgeons turned to minimally invasive techniques to adequately visualize and access the fetal trachea without a large hysterotomy. Fetal endoscopic (Fetendo) tracheal clipping, first performed in a human fetus in 1997, involved a maternal laparotomy, followed by 4 trocars through the maternal uterus to access and clip the fetal trachea.[80] Owing to complications of tracheal damage and vocal cord paralysis related to clipping, this technique evolved to the use of fetoscopic balloon tracheal occlusion, which avoids fetal neck dissection and requires only 1 uterine port (**Fig. 6**).[81]

Fetal endoscopic tracheal occlusion (FETO) is generally performed between 26 and 30 weeks of gestation. Under ultrasound guidance, a trocar is placed through the maternal abdomen into the amniotic cavity, and a fetoscope is inserted through the fetal mouth, and advanced into the fetal trachea. Once the carina has been visualized, the balloon is deployed by inflating it with physiologic solution just proximal to the carina. The correct placement is confirmed on ultrasound imaging and the instruments are removed.[68] In initial studies, the tracheal balloon was removed at the time of delivery via ex utero intrapartum therapy. However, balloon removal before birth not only allows for the possibility of vaginal birth, but also, in a fetal lamb model, was shown to increase type II pneumocyte differentiation, thereby increasing surfactant production.[82] Currently, tracheal occlusion is reversed in utero, by a second fetoscopic procedure typically at 34 weeks of gestation.[68]

A multicenter European series of 210 cases of FETO in singleton pregnancies with severe CDH (liver up and lung-to-head ratio ≤ 1) found a 48.0% rate of survival to discharge, with a 47.1% incidence of PPROM. When CDH registry data were used to compare outcomes with expectantly managed fetuses, FETO increased survival from 24.1% to 49.1% in fetuses with left CDH, and from 0% to 35.3% in right CDH.[83] A recent metaanalysis of all studies comparing survival outcome between FETO and a contemporary control group found that FETO improves survival compared with standard perinatal care in patients with isolated CDH and severe isolated pulmonary hypoplasia (lung-to-head ratio ≤ 1). Fifty-one of 110 fetuses (46.3%) who had undergone FETO survived to discharge, compared with 6 of 101 (5.9%) in the control group, giving the FETO group a significant survival advantage (odds ratio, 13.32; 95% CI, 5.40–32.87).[84] The true benefits of FETO are

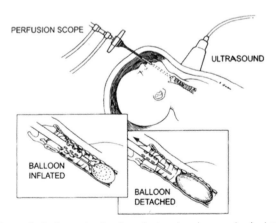

Fig. 6. Fetal endoscopic balloon tracheal occlusion involves a single intrauterine trocar, through which a fetoscope is introduced into the fetal trachea. A balloon is inflated just proximal to the carina.

difficult to gauge from these studies, because the severity of CDH was not measured uniformly and there was great variability in the postnatal care of these infants. An international, randomized trial to further evaluate the role of fetal therapy in patients with moderate and severe pulmonary hypoplasia (TOTAL trial, www. totaltrial.eu) is ongoing.[85]

Amniotic Band Syndrome

Amniotic band syndrome is a congenital malformation with a broad spectrum of clinical features. The presentation, severity, and outcome depend on location of the bands and timing of fetal damage.[86–88] Constriction bands at the extremities can lead to pseudosyndactyly or limb amputation (**Fig. 7**), whereas more midline bands can result in craniofacial, thoracic, or abdominal defects, and may be fatal. The etiology of this syndrome is unknown, and theories range from a genetic basis[89] or early disruption of the germinal disc[87,90] to traumatic disruption of the membranes later in fetal development.[91]

In cases of amniotic band syndrome with extremity involvement, fetoscopic band release may salvage normal development and allow the fetus to maintain limb function.[92–95] Diagnosis is made on obstetric ultrasound imaging, with findings including distal limb edema and abnormal Doppler flow, with or without visualization of the causative band. Although only small case series have been reported, the limited data suggest that fetuses must have abnormal but present arterial Doppler flow to the distal limb to benefit from intervention.[94] Moreover, data from our institution demonstrate that patients with single limb involvement tend to fare better than those with multiple involved limbs.[95] Interestingly, rates of PROM with this procedure seem to be higher than for other fetoscopic procedures, with reported rates up to 78%.[93] Although this finding may be related to the small number of cases and the learning curve required with any new procedure, it could also be a byproduct of the inherent membrane problems in these fetuses.[93]

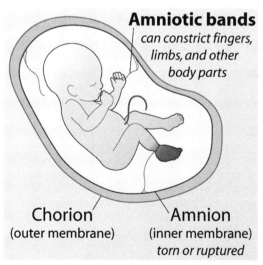

Fig. 7. Amniotic bands may constrict fetal limbs, leading to pseudosyndactyly or limb amputation. More midline bands can result in craniofacial, thoracic, or abdominal defects, and may be fatal.

Sacrococcygeal Teratoma

Fetuses with prenatally diagnosed sacrococcygeal teratoma (SCT) are at risk for perinatal complications and death, often owing to high-output cardiac failure. Fetal surgery has been proposed for SCT when hydrops and/or cardiac insufficiency are present in utero, particularly at previable gestational ages.[96] Open fetal surgery has been described, but is associated with a high risk of PPROM and preterm delivery.[97,98] Minimally invasive procedures for SCT focus on interrupting blood flow to the lesion using a variety of techniques, including coiling, embolization, sclerotherapy, monopolar cautery, laser ablation, and RFA.

In a recent systematic review of 34 cases of minimally invasive fetal intervention for SCT from 1980 to 2013,[99] overall survival was 44% (14/32) and mean gestational age at delivery was 29.7 ± 4.0 weeks. Cardiac failure conferred a worse prognosis, with only 30% survival (6/20) in this cohort. A subsequent review sought to distinguish between methods of minimally invasive interventions, discriminating between "interstitial" interventions, in which the goal is direct tumor ablation, and "vascular" interventions, in which the target is the feeding vessel to the tumor.[100] Of the 33 cases reviewed, 11 were vascular and 22 were interstitial ablations. Survival was 63.6% (7/11) in the vascular ablation group and 40.9% (9/22) in the interstitial ablation group. The authors hypothesized that reducing the tumor blood supply slowly may be safer than causing tumor necrosis that could lead to hemorrhage into the tumor.

Given the extremely poor outcomes of fetuses with large SCTs and fetal hydrops before viability,[99,101] available data suggest that fetal intervention does confer a survival advantage. However, because SCT is rare, data are limited to small case series, and randomized trials are likely impossible. Long-term outcomes data are also lacking. Because these procedures are associated with significant risks, they should be reserved only for selected severe cases presenting with both high-output heart failure and fetal hydrops before it is safe to deliver, and should be performed only in specialized centers.[99]

Congenital Cystic Adenomatoid Malformations and Pleural Effusions

Congenital cystic adenomatoid malformations are benign intrapulmonary masses that are classified as either microcystic or macrocystic (≥1 cysts >5 mm). The prognosis is generally good, with many lesions regressing or becoming undetectable late in gestation, and most infants are asymptomatic at birth.[102,103] However, some fetuses present with a lesion large enough to cause a mass effect, which leads to heart and lung compression and pulmonary hypoplasia. The presence of hydrops predicts very poor prognosis, with mortality of up to 100% without prenatal intervention.[101,104] The cystic adenomatoid malformation volume ratio is a useful sonographic marker for risk of hydrops, and a high cystic adenomatoid malformation volume ratio (≥1.6–2.0) is often used as an indication for fetal intervention.[105–107] In recent years, maternal betamethasone has become the first-line treatment of choice for large microcystic congenital cystic adenomatoid malformations, with reduction of cystic adenomatoid malformation volume ratio and resolution of hydrops in more than 80%.[108,109] However, steroid therapy has not been effective in predominately macrocystic lesions. In lesions with a dominant macrocyst or pleural effusion, in utero drainage can relieve the mass effect of excess fluid to allow for pulmonary development.[110–112]

Indications and known complications of thoracoamniotic shunt placement are summarized in **Table 4**. In the largest series of thoracoamniotic shunt placement for congenital lung mass or pleural effusion to date, which consisted of 75 fetuses at Children's Hospital of Philadelphia, shunting resulted in a 55% decrease in congenital

Table 4
Indications for and complications of thoracoamniotic shunt placement

Indications	Complications
<32 weeks of gestation with macrocystic lung lesion or pleural effusion	Preterm delivery
	PPROM
Presence of hydrops or high risk for pulmonary hypoplasia (ie, mediastinal shift, significant heart or lung compression)	Obstruction
	Dislodgement
	Bleeding
	Chest wall deformation (↑ risk with younger gestational age)[113]
Reaccumulation after thoracocentesis	
Nonlethal karyotype	
Lack of significant anatomic abnormalities	
Infectious etiology excluded (in isolated pleural effusion)	

Abbreviation: PPROM, preterm prelabor rupture of membranes.

cystic adenomatoid malformation volume and complete drainage of pleural effusion in 27% of cases (partial drainage in the remaining 73% of effusions).[112] Hydrops resolved in 83% of fetuses (43/53) after shunting, and hydrops resolution was strongly correlated with survival. Survival to birth was 93% (70/75), median gestational age was 36 weeks, and overall long-term survival was 68% (51/75). Fifty-six percent of fetuses were delivered preterm (<37 weeks of gestation), at an average of 10 weeks after shunt placement. Survivors had a median duration of stay in the neonatal intensive care unit of 21 days, with 71% requiring intubation for greater than 24 hours. This series affirms the survival benefit of shunting in these high-risk patients, but underscores the risks inherent to in utero intervention, as well as the intensive neonatal therapy required.

FUTURE DIRECTIONS

The future of fetal therapy is undoubtedly moving toward minimally invasive treatment. As always, the goal of fetal therapy is to provide the best possible outcome for the fetus, while minimizing the risk to the mother. To this end, significant efforts are being made toward decreasing the morbidity associated with fetal intervention, particularly PPROM. A multiinstitution collaboration between University of California San Francisco, the University of California Berkeley, and Caltech is currently focusing on the development of a biocompatible adhesive to preseal amniotic membranes before fetal therapy to prevent PPROM (**Fig. 8**). Current formulations involve

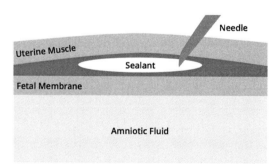

Fig. 8. A biocompatible adhesive, "Amnioseal" is currently under development, which can be delivered just below the uterus to preseal the fetal membrane before amniotic access.

methyldihydroxyphenylalanine-based polymers inspired by the adhesive properties of mussels' attachment to wet rocks.[114]

Although fetal surgical intervention is limited to the correction of structural anomalies, prenatal stem cell transplantation and gene therapy have the potential to treat a wide range of genetic conditions. The rationale for in utero stem cell transplantation is to take advantage of the process of normal immune development and introduce "foreign" cells before the fetus distinguishes self from non-self.[115] Currently, the most promising applications of fetal stem cell therapy for potential clinical use are in utero hematopoietic stem cell transplantation and in utero mesenchymal stem cell transplantation.[116] Clinical trials of in utero hematopoietic stem cell transplantation have had limited success in recipients without underlying immunodeficiency,[117] but recent experimental data in a large animal model of intrauterine hematopoietic stem cell transplantation have demonstrated clinically relevant levels of chimerism, supporting the path to clinical trials for inherited hematologic disorders.[118,119] In utero human fetal mesenchymal stem cell transplantation has been described for osteogenesis imperfecta with promising, but transient results.[120] Finally, fetal gene therapy also has exciting potential for the treatment of genetic disorders, and recent gene-editing technology such as CRISPR is significantly advancing the field. However, the safety and long-term effect of these therapies must be thoroughly investigated in animal models.[116,121]

REFERENCES

1. Harrison MR, Evans MI, Adzick NS, et al. The unborn patient: the art and science of fetal therapy. 3rd edition. Philadelphia: W.B. Saunders Company; 2001.

2. Liley AW. Intrauterine transfusion of foetus in haemolytic disease. Br Med J 1963;2:1107–9.

3. Pringle KC. Fetal surgery: it has a past, has it a future? Fetal Ther 1986;1:23–31.

4. Deprest JA, Flake AW, Gratacos E, et al. The making of fetal surgery. Prenat Diagn 2010;30:653–67.

5. Estes JM, MacGillivray TE, Hedrick MH, et al. Fetoscopic surgery for the treatment of congenital anomalies. J Pediatr Surg 1992;27:950–4.

6. Estes JM, Szabo Z, Harrison MR. Techniques for in utero endoscopic surgery. A new approach for fetal intervention. Surg Endosc 1992;6:215–8.

7. Luks FI, Deprest JA. Endoscopic fetal surgery: a new alternative? Eur J Obstet Gynecol Reprod Biol 1993;52:1–3.

8. Sydorak RM, Albanese CT. Minimal access techniques for fetal surgery. World J Surg 2003;27:95–102.

9. American College of Obstetricians and Gynecologists, Committee on Ethics, American Academy of Pediatrics, Committee on Bioethics. Maternal-fetal intervention and fetal care centers. Pediatrics 2011;128:e473–8.

10. Chervenak FA, McCullough LB. Ethics of fetal surgery. Clin Perinatol 2009;36:237–46, vii-viii.

11. Luks FI, Johnson A, Polzin WJ. Innovation in maternal-fetal therapy: a position statement from the North American Fetal Therapy Network. Obstet Gynecol 2015;125:649–52.

12. Lin EE, Tran KM. Anesthesia for fetal surgery. Semin Pediatr Surg 2013;22:50–5.

13. Deprest JA, Van Schoubroeck D, Van Ballaer PP, et al. Alternative technique for Nd:YAG laser coagulation in twin-to-twin transfusion syndrome with anterior placenta. Ultrasound Obstet Gynecol 1998;11:347–52.

14. Petersen SG, Gibbons KS, Luks FI, et al. The impact of entry technique and access diameter on prelabour rupture of membranes following primary fetoscopic laser treatment for twin-twin transfusion syndrome. Fetal Diagn Ther 2016;40: 100–9.

15. Van de Velde M, De Buck F. Fetal and maternal analgesia/anesthesia for fetal procedures. Fetal Diagn Ther 2012;31:201–9.

16. De Buck F, Deprest J, Van de Velde M. Anesthesia for fetal surgery. Curr Opin Anaesthesiol 2008;21:293–7.

17. Sviggum HP, Kodali BS. Maternal anesthesia for fetal surgery. Clin Perinatol 2013;40:413–27.

18. Beck V, Lewi P, Gucciardo L, et al. Preterm prelabor rupture of membranes and fetal survival after minimally invasive fetal surgery: a systematic review of the literature. Fetal Diagn Ther 2012;31:1–9.

19. Snowise S, Mann LK, Moise KJ Jr, et al. Preterm prelabor rupture of membranes after fetoscopic laser surgery for twin-twin transfusion syndrome. Ultrasound Obstet Gynecol 2017;49:607–11.

20. Kohl T. Percutaneous minimally invasive fetoscopic surgery for spina bifida aperta. Part I: surgical technique and perioperative outcome. Ultrasound Obstet Gynecol 2014;44:515–24.

21. Degenhardt J, Schurg R, Winarno A, et al. Percutaneous minimal-access fetoscopic surgery for spina bifida aperta. Part II: maternal management and outcome. Ultrasound Obstet Gynecol 2014;44:525–31.

22. Graf K, Kohl T, Neubauer BA, et al. Percutaneous minimally invasive fetoscopic surgery for spina bifida aperta. Part III: neurosurgical intervention in the first postnatal year. Ultrasound Obstet Gynecol 2016;47:158–61.

23. Pedreira DA, Zanon N, Nishikuni K, et al. Endoscopic surgery for the antenatal treatment of myelomeningocele: the CECAM trial. Am J Obstet Gynecol 2016; 214:111.e111.

24. Farrell JA, Albanese CT, Jennings RW, et al. Maternal fertility is not affected by fetal surgery. Fetal Diagn Ther 1999;14:190–2.

25. Wilson RD, Lemerand K, Johnson MP, et al. Reproductive outcomes in subsequent pregnancies after a pregnancy complicated by open maternal-fetal surgery (1996-2007). Am J Obstet Gynecol 2010;203:209.e1-6.

26. Johnson A. Diagnosis and management of twin-twin transfusion syndrome. Clin Obstet Gynecol 2015;58:611–31.

27. Behrendt N, Galan HL. Twin-twin transfusion and laser therapy. Curr Opin Obstet Gynecol 2016;28:79–85.

28. Quintero RA, Morales WJ, Allen MH, et al. Staging of twin-twin transfusion syndrome. J Perinatol 1999;19:550–5.

29. Senat MV, Deprest J, Boulvain M, et al. Endoscopic laser surgery versus serial amnioreduction for severe twin-to-twin transfusion syndrome. N Engl J Med 2004;351:136–44.

30. Roberts D, Neilson JP, Kilby MD, et al. Interventions for the treatment of twin-twin transfusion syndrome. Cochrane Database Syst Rev 2014;(1):CD002073.

31. Rossi AC, D'Addario V. Laser therapy and serial amnioreduction as treatment for twin-twin transfusion syndrome: a metaanalysis and review of literature. Am J Obstet Gynecol 2008;198:147–52.

32. De Lia JE, Cruikshank DP, Keye WR Jr. Fetoscopic neodymium:YAG laser occlusion of placental vessels in severe twin-twin transfusion syndrome. Obstet Gynecol 1990;75:1046–53.

33. Crombleholme TM, Shera D, Lee H, et al. A prospective, randomized, multi-center trial of amnioreduction vs selective fetoscopic laser photocoagulation for the treatment of severe twin-twin transfusion syndrome. Am J Obstet Gynecol 2007;197:396.e1-9.

34. Emery SP, Hasley SK, Catov JM, et al. North American Fetal Therapy Network: intervention vs expectant management for stage I twin-twin transfusion syndrome. Am J Obstet Gynecol 2016;215:346.e1-7.

35. Trevett T, Johnson A. Monochorionic twin pregnancies. Clin Perinatol 2005;32: 475–94, viii.

36. Peng R, Xie HN, Lin MF, et al. Clinical outcomes after selective fetal reduction of complicated monochorionic twins with radiofrequency ablation and bipolar cord coagulation. Gynecol Obstet Invest 2016;81:552–8.

37. Ong SS, Zamora J, Khan KS, et al. Prognosis for the co-twin following single-twin death: a systematic review. BJOG 2006;113:992–8.

38. Yinon Y, Ashwal E, Weisz B, et al. Selective reduction in complicated mono-chorionic twins: prediction of obstetric outcome and comparison of tech-niques. Ultrasound Obstet Gynecol 2015;46:670–7.

39. Lee H, Bebbington M, Crombleholme TM. The North American Fetal Therapy Network Registry data on outcomes of radiofrequency ablation for twin-reversed arterial perfusion sequence. Fetal Diagn Ther 2013;33:224–9.

40. Farrugia MK. Fetal bladder outlet obstruction: embryopathology, in utero inter-vention and outcome. J Pediatr Urol 2016;12:296–303.

41. Ruano R, Duarte S, Bunduki V, et al. Fetal cystoscopy for severe lower urinary tract obstruction–initial experience of a single center. Prenat Diagn 2010;30: 30–9.

42. Kilby M, Khan K, Morris K, et al. PLUTO trial protocol: percutaneous shunting for lower urinary tract obstruction randomised controlled trial. BJOG 2007;114: 904–5, e1-4.

43. Matsell DG, Yu S, Morrison SJ. Antenatal determinants of long-term kidney outcome in boys with posterior urethral valves. Fetal Diagn Ther 2016;39: 214–21.

44. Harrison MR, Nakayama DK, Noall R, et al. Correction of congenital hydroneph-rosis in utero II. Decompression reverses the effects of obstruction on the fetal lung and urinary tract. J Pediatr Surg 1982;17:965–74.

45. Farrugia MK, Long DA, Godley ML, et al. Experimental short-term fetal bladder outflow obstruction: I. Morphology and cell biology associated with urinary flow impairment. J Pediatr Urol 2006;2:243–53.

46. Peters CA, Carr MC, Lais A, et al. The response of the fetal kidney to obstruc-tion. J Urol 1992;148:503–9.

47. Harrison MR, Golbus MS, Filly RA, et al. Management of the fetus with congen-ital hydronephrosis. J Pediatr Surg 1982;17:728–42.

48. Harrison MR, Ross N, Noall R, et al. Correction of congenital hydronephrosis in utero. I. The model: fetal urethral obstruction produces hydronephrosis and pul-monary hypoplasia in fetal lambs. J Pediatr Surg 1983;18:247–56.

49. Harrison MR, Golbus MS, Filly RA, et al. Fetal surgery for congenital hydroneph-rosis. N Engl J Med 1982;306:591–3.

50. Smith-Harrison LI, Hougen HY, Timberlake MD, et al. Current applications of in utero intervention for lower urinary tract obstruction. J Pediatr Urol 2015;11: 341–7.

51. Clark TJ, Martin WL, Divakaran TG, et al. Prenatal bladder drainage in the management of fetal lower urinary tract obstruction: a systematic review and meta-analysis. Obstet Gynecol 2003;102:367–82.

52. Morris RK, Malin GL, Quinlan-Jones E, et al. Percutaneous vesicoamniotic shunting versus conservative management for fetal lower urinary tract obstruction (PLUTO): a randomised trial. Lancet 2013;382:1496–506.

53. Ruano R, Sananes N, Sangi-Haghpeykar H, et al. Fetal intervention for severe lower urinary tract obstruction: a multicenter case-control study comparing fetal cystoscopy with vesicoamniotic shunting. Ultrasound Obstet Gynecol 2015;45: 452–8.

54. Sananes N, Cruz-Martinez R, Favre R, et al. Two-year outcomes after diagnostic and therapeutic fetal cystoscopy for lower urinary tract obstruction. Prenat Diagn 2016;36:297–303.

55. Saadai P, Farmer DL. Fetal surgery for myelomeningocele. Clin Perinatol 2012; 39:279–88.

56. Meuli M, Meuli-Simmen C, Hutchins GM, et al. The spinal cord lesion in human fetuses with myelomeningocele: implications for fetal surgery. J Pediatr Surg 1997;32:448–52.

57. Meuli M, Meuli-Simmen C, Yingling CD, et al. Creation of myelomeningocele in utero: a model of functional damage from spinal cord exposure in fetal sheep. J Pediatr Surg 1995;30:1028–32 [discussion: 1032–3].

58. Paek BW, Farmer DL, Wilkinson CC, et al. Hindbrain herniation develops in surgically created myelomeningocele but is absent after repair in fetal lambs. Am J Obstet Gynecol 2000;183:1119–23.

59. Yoshizawa J, Sbragia L, Paek BW, et al. Fetal surgery for repair of myelomeningocele allows normal development of the rectum in sheep. Pediatr Surg Int 2003;19:162–6.

60. Meuli M, Meuli-Simmen C, Yingling CD, et al. In utero repair of experimental myelomeningocele saves neurological function at birth. J Pediatr Surg 1996; 31:397–402.

61. Adzick NS. Fetal surgery for spina bifida: past, present, future. Semin Pediatr Surg 2013;22:10–7.

62. Bruner JP, Tulipan NE, Richards WO. Endoscopic coverage of fetal open myelomeningocele in utero. Am J Obstet Gynecol 1997;176:256–7.

63. Bruner JP, Richards WO, Tulipan NB, et al. Endoscopic coverage of fetal myelomeningocele in utero. Am J Obstet Gynecol 1999;180:153–8.

64. Adzick NS, Sutton LN, Crombleholme TM, et al. Successful fetal surgery for spina bifida. Lancet 1998;352:1675–6.

65. Bruner JP, Tulipan N, Paschall RL, et al. Fetal surgery for myelomeningocele and the incidence of shunt-dependent hydrocephalus. JAMA 1999;282:1819–25.

66. Adzick NS, Thom EA, Spong CY, et al. A randomized trial of prenatal versus postnatal repair of myelomeningocele. N Engl J Med 2011;364:993–1004.

67. Flake A. Percutaneous minimal-access fetoscopic surgery for myelomeningocele - not so minimal! Ultrasound Obstet Gynecol 2014;44:499–500.

68. Ruano R, Ali RA, Patel P, et al. Fetal endoscopic tracheal occlusion for congenital diaphragmatic hernia: indications, outcomes, and future directions. Obstet Gynecol Surv 2014;69:147–58.

69. Done E, Gratacos E, Nicolaides KH, et al. Predictors of neonatal morbidity in fetuses with severe isolated congenital diaphragmatic hernia undergoing fetoscopic tracheal occlusion. Ultrasound Obstet Gynecol 2013;42:77–83.

70. Shue EH, Miniati D, Lee H. Advances in prenatal diagnosis and treatment of congenital diaphragmatic hernia. Clin Perinatol 2012;39:289–300.
71. Harrison MR, Adzick NS, Flake AW, et al. Correction of congenital diaphragmatic hernia in utero: VI. Hard-earned lessons. J Pediatr Surg 1993;28:1411–7 [discussion: 1417–8].
72. Harrison MR, Adzick NS, Bullard KM, et al. Correction of congenital diaphragmatic hernia in utero VII: a prospective trial. J Pediatr Surg 1997;32:1637–42.
73. Hedrick MH, Ferro MM, Filly RA, et al. Congenital high airway obstruction syndrome (CHAOS): a potential for perinatal intervention. J Pediatr Surg 1994;29:271–4.
74. DiFiore JW, Fauza DO, Slavin R, et al. Experimental fetal tracheal ligation reverses the structural and physiological effects of pulmonary hypoplasia in congenital diaphragmatic hernia. J Pediatr Surg 1994;29:248–56 [discussion: 256–7].
75. Hedrick MH, Estes JM, Sullivan KM, et al. Plug the lung until it grows (PLUG): a new method to treat congenital diaphragmatic hernia in utero. J Pediatr Surg 1994;29:612–7.
76. Bealer JF, Skarsgard ED, Hedrick MH, et al. The 'PLUG' odyssey: adventures in experimental fetal tracheal occlusion. J Pediatr Surg 1995;30:361–4 [discussion: 364–5].
77. Kitano Y, Davies P, von Allmen D, et al. Fetal tracheal occlusion in the rat model of nitrogen-induced congenital diaphragmatic hernia. J Appl Physiol (1985) 1999;87:769–75.
78. Kitano Y, Kanai M, Davies P, et al. BAPS prize-1999: lung growth induced by prenatal tracheal occlusion and its modifying factors: a study in the rat model of congenital diaphragmatic hernia. J Pediatr Surg 2001;36:251–9.
79. Harrison MR, Adzick NS, Flake AW, et al. Correction of congenital diaphragmatic hernia in utero VIII: response of the hypoplastic lung to tracheal occlusion. J Pediatr Surg 1996;31:1339–48.
80. VanderWall KJ, Skarsgard ED, Filly RA, et al. Fetendo-clip: a fetal endoscopic tracheal clip procedure in a human fetus. J Pediatr Surg 1997;32:970–2.
81. Harrison MR, Albanese CT, Hawgood SB, et al. Fetoscopic temporary tracheal occlusion by means of detachable balloon for congenital diaphragmatic hernia. Am J Obstet Gynecol 2001;185:730–3.
82. Bin Saddiq W, Piedboeuf B, Laberge JM, et al. The effects of tracheal occlusion and release on type II pneumocytes in fetal lambs. J Pediatr Surg 1997;32:834–8.
83. Jani JC, Nicolaides KH, Gratacos E, et al. Severe diaphragmatic hernia treated by fetal endoscopic tracheal occlusion. Ultrasound Obstet Gynecol 2009;34:304–10.
84. Al-Maary J, Eastwood MP, Russo FM, et al. Fetal tracheal occlusion for severe pulmonary hypoplasia in isolated congenital diaphragmatic hernia: a systematic review and meta-analysis of survival. Ann Surg 2016;264:929–33.
85. Deprest J, De Coppi P. Antenatal management of isolated congenital diaphragmatic hernia today and tomorrow: ongoing collaborative research and development. Journal of Pediatric Surgery Lecture. J Pediatr Surg 2012;47:282–90.
86. Seeds JW, Cefalo RC, Herbert WN. Amniotic band syndrome. Am J Obstet Gynecol 1982;144:243–8.
87. Bamforth JS. Amniotic band sequence: Streeter's hypothesis reexamined. Am J Med Genet 1992;44:280–7.
88. Iqbal CW, Derderian SC, Cheng Y, et al. Amniotic band syndrome: a single-institutional experience. Fetal Diagn Ther 2015;37:1–5.

89. Cignini P, Giorlandino C, Padula F, et al. Epidemiology and risk factors of amniotic band syndrome, or ADAM sequence. J Prenat Med 2012;6:59–63.

90. Bamforth JS. Amniotic band sequence: Streeter's hypothesis reexamined. Am J Med Genet 1992;44:280–7.

91. Torpin R. Amniochorionic mesoblastic fibrous strings and amniotic bands: associated constricting fetal malformations or fetal death. Am J Obstet Gynecol 1965;91:65–75.

92. Quintero RA, Morales WJ, Phillips J, et al. In utero lysis of amniotic bands. Ultrasound Obstet Gynecol 1997;10:316–20.

93. Richter J, Wergeland H, DeKoninck P, et al. Fetoscopic release of an amniotic band with risk of amputation: case report and review of the literature. Fetal Diagn Ther 2012;31:134–7.

94. Husler MR, Wilson RD, Horii SC, et al. When is fetoscopic release of amniotic bands indicated? Review of outcome of cases treated in utero and selection criteria for fetal surgery. Prenat Diagn 2009;29:457–63.

95. Derderian SC, Iqbal CW, Goldstein R, et al. Fetoscopic approach to amniotic band syndrome. J Pediatr Surg 2014;49:359–62.

96. Kitagawa H, Pringle KC. Fetal surgery: a critical review. Pediatr Surg Int 2017; 33(4):421–33.

97. Adzick NS, Crombleholme TM, Morgan MA, et al. A rapidly growing fetal teratoma. Lancet 1997;349:538.

98. Hedrick HL, Flake AW, Crombleholme TM, et al. Sacrococcygeal teratoma: prenatal assessment, fetal intervention, and outcome. J Pediatr Surg 2004;39: 430–8 [discussion: 430–8].

99. Van Mieghem T, Al-Ibrahim A, Deprest J, et al. Minimally invasive therapy for fetal sacrococcygeal teratoma: case series and systematic review of the literature. Ultrasound Obstet Gynecol 2014;43:611–9.

100. Sananes N, Javadian P, Schwach Werneck Britto I, et al. Technical aspects and effectiveness of percutaneous fetal therapies for large sacrococcygeal teratomas: cohort study and literature review. Ultrasound Obstet Gynecol 2016; 47:712–9.

101. Grethel EJ, Wagner AJ, Clifton MS, et al. Fetal intervention for mass lesions and hydrops improves outcome: a 15-year experience. J Pediatr Surg 2007;42: 117–23.

102. Baird R, Puligandla PS, Laberge JM. Congenital lung malformations: informing best practice. Semin Pediatr Surg 2014;23:270–7.

103. Kunisaki SM, Ehrenberg-Buchner S, Dillman JR, et al. Vanishing fetal lung malformations: prenatal sonographic characteristics and postnatal outcomes. J Pediatr Surg 2015;50:978–82.

104. Adzick NS, Harrison MR, Crombleholme TM, et al. Fetal lung lesions: management and outcome. Am J Obstet Gynecol 1998;179:884–9.

105. Crombleholme TM, Coleman B, Hedrick H, et al. Cystic adenomatoid malformation volume ratio predicts outcome in prenatally diagnosed cystic adenomatoid malformation of the lung. J Pediatr Surg 2002;37:331–8.

106. Cass DL, Olutoye OO, Cassady CI, et al. Prenatal diagnosis and outcome of fetal lung masses. J Pediatr Surg 2011;46:292–8.

107. Ehrenberg-Buchner S, Stapf AM, Berman DR, et al. Fetal lung lesions: can we start to breathe easier? Am J Obstet Gynecol 2013;208:151.e1-7.

108. Peranteau WH, Boelig MM, Khalek N, et al. Effect of single and multiple courses of maternal betamethasone on prenatal congenital lung lesion growth and fetal survival. J Pediatr Surg 2016;51:28–32.

109. Curran PF, Jelin EB, Rand L, et al. Prenatal steroids for microcystic congenital cystic adenomatoid malformations. J Pediatr Surg 2010;45:145–50.
110. Nicolaides KH, Blott M, Greenough A. Chronic drainage of fetal pulmonary cyst. Lancet 1987;1:618.
111. Wilson RD, Baxter JK, Johnson MP, et al. Thoracoamniotic shunts: fetal treatment of pleural effusions and congenital cystic adenomatoid malformations. Fetal Diagn Ther 2004;19:413–20.
112. Peranteau WH, Adzick NS, Boelig MM, et al. Thoracoamniotic shunts for the management of fetal lung lesions and pleural effusions: a single-institution review and predictors of survival in 75 cases. J Pediatr Surg 2015;50:301–5.
113. Merchant AM, Peranteau W, Wilson RD, et al. Postnatal chest wall deformities after fetal thoracoamniotic shunting for congenital cystic adenomatoid malformation. Fetal Diagn Ther 2007;22:435–9.
114. Graves CE, Arun A, Lee J, et al. Amnioseal: biomimetic adhesives to preseal fetal membranes for prevention of PPROM after fetal intervention. Paper presented at: World Federation of Associations of Pediatric Surgeons Congress 2016; Washington, DC.
115. Keller BA, Hirose S, Farmer DL. Fetal therapy. In: Milunsky A, editor. Genetic disorders and the fetus: diagnosis, prevention, and treatment. 7th edition. Hoboken (NJ): John Wiley & Sons, Inc.; 2016. p. 989–1011.
116. McClain LE, Flake AW. In utero stem cell transplantation and gene therapy: recent progress and the potential for clinical application. Best Pract Res Clin Obstet Gynaecol 2016;31:88–98.
117. Flake AW, Zanjani ED. In utero hematopoietic stem cell transplantation: ontogenic opportunities and biologic barriers. Blood 1999;94:2179–91.
118. Vrecenak JD, Pearson EG, Santore MT, et al. Stable long-term mixed chimerism achieved in a canine model of allogeneic in utero hematopoietic cell transplantation. Blood 2014;124:1987–95.
119. MacKenzie TC. Fetal Surgical conditions and the unraveling of maternal-fetal tolerance. J Pediatr Surg 2016;51:197–9.
120. Chan JK, Gotherstrom C. Prenatal transplantation of mesenchymal stem cells to treat osteogenesis imperfecta. Front Pharmacol 2014;5:223.
121. MacKenzie TC, David AL, Flake AW, et al. Consensus statement from the first international conference for in utero stem cell transplantation and gene therapy. Front Pharmacol 2015;6:15.

Esophageal Atresia and Upper Airway Pathology

David C. van der Zee, MD, PhD*, Maud Y.A. van Herwaarden, MD, PhD,
Caroline C. Hulsker, MD, Marieke J. Witvliet, MD,
Stefaan H.A. Tytgat, MD, PhD

KEYWORDS

- Esophageal atresia • Long gap esophageal atresia • Tracheoesophageal fistula
- Esophageal stenosis • Tracheomalacia • Recurrent fistula
- Gastroesophageal reflux disease

KEY POINTS

- Esophageal atresia is an anomaly with frequently occurring sequelae requiring lifelong management and follow-up.
- There is an increasing awareness of the anesthetic and surgical implications in the care of neonates with esophageal atresia.
- Because of the complex issues encountered, patients with esophageal atresia preferably should be managed in centers of expertise.

INTRODUCTION

With improved neonatal care focus in esophageal atresia, the current focus in outcomes has shifted from mortality to morbidity. Esophageal atresia is not merely a congenital malformation that warrants surgical treatment but is an anomaly with frequently occurring sequelae requiring lifelong management and follow-up.[1] The pediatric surgeon may play a key role in the management of children born with esophageal atresia, which implies not only using advanced techniques to restore continuity but also providing optimal perinatal care and follow-up into adulthood. In a recent publication from the European Society for Pediatric Gastroenterology, Hepatology, and Nutrition–North American Society for Pediatric Gastroenterology, a joint article from the European and North American pediatric gastroenterology societies, guidelines were presented for the evaluation and treatment of gastrointestinal and nutritional complications in children with esophageal atresia.[1]

Disclosure Statement: The authors have nothing to disclose.
Department of Pediatric Surgery, University Medical Center Utrecht, KE. 04.140.5, PO Box 85090, Utrecht 3508 AB, The Netherlands
* Corresponding author.
E-mail address: d.c.vanderzee@umcutrecht.nl

Clin Perinatol 44 (2017) 753–762
http://dx.doi.org/10.1016/j.clp.2017.08.002
0095-5108/17/© 2017 Elsevier Inc. All rights reserved.
perinatology.theclinics.com

In addition to paying more attention to follow-up, there is an increasing awareness of the anesthetic and surgical implications in the care of these newborns. Disquieting reports have recently been published on the possible negative effects on neurodevelopment in children born with noncardiac major congenital anomalies.[2,3] Perinatal brain monitoring has become a major issue in managing this cohort of patients.[4–7]

The Department of Pediatric Surgery at the University Medical Center in Utrecht is a center recognized by the government for the authors' expertise in esophageal atresia and upper airway management. Patients are referred from throughout the country and abroad for specific management or reiterative surgery and airway problems. Results were recently published.[8] This article describes the management of minimally invasive surgery in esophageal atresia and upper airway pathology.

PRENATAL DIAGNOSIS

Prenatal symptoms may be polyhydramnios detected on physical examination or ultrasound.[9,10] Routinely performed ultrasound during pregnancy may show regurgitation of amniotic fluid during swallowing or the absence of gastric contents, in particular in patients with type A atresia with no fistula.[9–12] Antenatal MRI has a high sensitivity for the confirmation of esophageal atresia.[10,12,13] The sensitivity is significantly higher in high-level fetal centers.[10,13]

POSTNATAL DIAGNOSIS AND WORKUP

There are principally 6 types of esophageal anomalies (**Fig. 1**). The most common sign of esophageal atresia is the inability to advance a nasogastric tube during postnatal care. Usually a plain thoracic and abdominal radiogram will show the curling of the nasogastric tube in the proximal esophagus. Additionally, air in the stomach and intestines indicates the presence of a distal fistula, whereas the absence of air indicates isolated esophageal atresia. On establishing the diagnosis, patients are admitted into the neonatal intensive care unit (NICU) and are given an intravenous (IV) drip, an arterial line, and a orogastric tube to empty the proximal esophagus (**Box 1**). Nowadays, all neonates have near-infrared spectrometry and α-electroencephalogram (EEG) to monitor brain oxygenation. Further immediate workup consists of consultation of the pediatric cardiologist to determine cardiac malformations and locate the side of the descending aorta as well as the performance of an ultrasound of kidneys and brain. Consultation of a geneticist, an ophthalmologist, and other pediatric specialists depending on concomitant anomalies are performed as necessary.

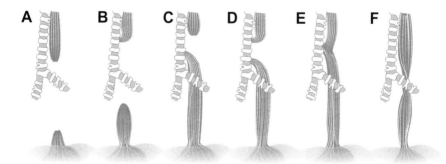

Fig. 1. Six types of esophageal atresia: type A, no fistula; type B, proximal fistula; type C, distal fistula; type D, both proximal and distal fistula; type E, only fistula; type F, esophageal stenosis.

Box 1
Protocol patients with esophageal atresia

Summary workup on admission in NICU

- Preoperative workup
  - IV drip, arterial line, laboratory tests
  - Replogle tube drainage
  - Near-infrared spectrometry, a-EEG
  - Consultation pediatric cardiologist + echocardiogram
  - Radiogram-thorax/abdomen, ultrasound kidneys
  - Consultation genetics
  - Consultation ophthalmologist
  - Other investigations depending on concomitant anomalies

- Preoperative multidisciplinary consultation on intended procedure

- After induction, preoperative rigid trachea-bronchoscopy

- Operative thoracoscopic correction esophageal atresia under near-infrared spectrometry and a-EEG control

- Postoperative ventilation for 24 to 48 hours on indication

- Start ranitidine

- Start feeding through nasogastric tube after 24 hours

- Start oral feeding or breast feeding when no saliva and/or infectious symptoms

- Transfer to ward when stable and spontaneous breathing

- MRI brain after 1 week

- Life support course parents

- Discharge from hospital when on full enteral feeds and no other sequelae

---

There is a preoperative multidisciplinary meeting with all involved specialists, that is, neonatologist, pediatric anesthesiologist, pediatric ear, nose, and throat specialist, pediatric surgeon, and, if necessary, pediatric cardiologist.

PREOPERATIVE RIGID TRACHEOSCOPY

An important step for management is the preoperative rigid tracheoscopy with spontaneous breathing.[14] The indication is twofold: (1) to determine the presence and level of the distal fistula in relation to the tracheal bifurcation. If deemed difficult to find during surgery, even a small catheter or guidewire can be inserted to make finding the fistula easier. Also important in using a rigid bronchoscope is to exclude a proximal fistula. The proximal fistula may be difficult to see; by scraping backward with the rigid tracheoscope over the posterior wall, a proximal fistula may open up and (2) to determine the presence and extent of tracheomalacia.[15] Tracheomalacia may occur because of insufficiency of the tracheal rings and/or a floppy pars membranacea. In normal circumstances, the pars membranacea forms approximately one-third of the circumference of the trachea. In children with esophageal atresia, this may increase to 50% or even more. During expiration, the positive intrathoracic pressure may push up the pars membranacea against the anterior wall of the trachea. Sometimes the distal fistula will hold back the pars membranacea, but by transecting the fistula the floppy pars membranacea is no longer restrained and may close up the tracheal space postoperatively.

OPERATIVE PROCEDURE

The authors' department has operated on all patients thoracoscopically since 2000. The procedure was described extensively before and is only summarized here.[14,16–18]

Proximal Fistula

Depending on the level of the proximal fistula, this may be approached from the neck on the right side in high fistula before the thoracoscopy. From an approach anterior to the sternocleidomastoid muscle, the esophagus can be identified and mobilized. The recurrent nerve is identified. Superior and caudal to the tracheoesophageal fistula, a vessel loop can be introduced and the fistula can be further dissected. The tracheal side can be closed by a transfixing suture, before cutting the fistula. The esophageal side can then be closed with interrupted sutures.[19]

If the proximal fistula can be approached thoracoscopically, it can be managed in the same procedure as the anastomosis of the esophagus.

Thoracoscopic Repair of Esophageal Atresia with Distal Fistula

The child is placed in a three-quarter left prone position at the left side of the operating table. A 5-mm trocar is placed approximately 1 cm inferior and anterior to the scapula tip for the camera. Two 3-mm trocars are placed under direct vision in a triangle around the 5-mm trocar for instrumentation. Insufflation is started at 3 to 5 mm Hg with a flow of 1 L/min. There is close collaboration with the anesthesiologist to maintain patients on an adequate saturation level both by oxygen saturation and near-infrared spectrometry of the brain circulation. Usually the ventilation frequency is increased up to 50 to 60/min while maintaining the same minute volume. Only when everyone is satisfied, the anesthesiologist with the ventilation and the pediatric surgeon with the desufflation of the right lung, the procedure can be started. Usually the first step is to mobilize the distal esophagus. The distal esophagus can be found by following the anterior vagal nerve distally. The pleura can be incised superior to the vagal nerve approximately 1 cm inferior to the azygos vein. After having mobilized the esophagus circumferentially, the entry into the tracheal wall can be dissected and ligated. Depending on the level of the fistula, the azygos vein is taken down to give more access to the entry point of the fistula into the trachea. Some investigators prefer to maintain the azygos vein, but there is no absolute indication. After sufficient mobilization of the distal esophagus, the pleura over the proximal esophagus is opened. The proximal esophagus can be identified by having the anesthesiologist push on the orogastric tube in the proximal esophagus. This moment is also the time to dissect a proximal fistula if one exists, under identification of the anterior and posterior vagal nerve. Management of a proximal fistula is similar to the cervical procedure. Finally, after opening the proximal esophagus, an end-to-end anastomosis can be made. A transanastomotic tube is left behind to start early feeding. There is no scientific evidence that interposition of tissue will preclude recurrence of a fistula. No pleural drainage is left behind.

Thoracoscopic Repair of Long Gap Esophageal Atresia

In cases of a long gap esophageal atresia, primary anastomosis is not possible. Recently, a working group of the International Network of Esophageal Atresia published a definition of long gap esophageal atresia as: any type of esophageal atresia in which there is no abdominal air on plain abdominal radiograph, which implies type A and B esophageal atresia.[20] All other types may be difficult to make an anastomosis but are not considered a long gap. There are several ways to deal with a long gap esophageal atresia. The currently most-often applied approach is a delayed primary anastomosis, which means that patients receive an orogastric tube in the proximal esophagus to clear salivation and a gastrostomy for feeding. Then after 2 to 4 months, an attempt is made to undertake a primary anastomosis.[21,22] If the distance is still too large, substitution may be considered by gastric pull-up, jejunal interposition, or colon interposition.[23–27] In the authors' institution, they have gained much experience with thoracoscopic procedures and have started a program in which traction sutures are applied on both ends of the esophagus after elaborate thoracoscopic mobilization.[17] Within the next days, the 2 ends approach each other and a primary anastomosis can be undertaken. Initially the patients were given a gastrostomy for feeding, and the procedure was delayed until referral to the authors' unit. Nowadays principally the patients are operated on within the first week of life without a gastrostomy, although a laparoscopic gastropexy is performed to prevent the stomach from migrating into the thorax. Usually after 4 to 6 days the ends have approached each other sufficiently to make a thoracoscopic primary anastomosis. If after 5 days the contrast study shows no leakage, the neonates can start oral feeding; depending on their maturity and concomitant anomalies, they can go home after 3 to 4 weeks.

Thoracoscopic Repair of Congenital Esophageal Stenosis

The congenital esophageal stenosis is usually located in the distal esophagus and may be best approached from the left side with patients in a supine position in which the table can be tilted into an appropriate position. A higher position of the stenosis may be approached from the right side.[18] The technique is similar to the earlier described procedures. By introducing a balloon catheter into the esophagus and inflating the balloon distally from the stenosis, the exact location of the stenosis can be determined. Sometimes simultaneous esophagoscopy is of use to determine the exact location of the stenosis. The procedure performed depends on the type of tissue encountered. In case of a cartilage ring, a circular resection of the stenosis is necessary with end-to-end anastomosis. The anterior and posterior vagal nerves are dissected from the esophageal wall and should be preserved. In case of fibrous tissue, a longitudinal incision can be made with transverse closure of the defect to widen the stenosis. A transanastomotic tube is left behind for early feeding.

Thoracoscopic Approach for Life-Threatening Events in Tracheomalacia

The most frequently used technique for alleviation of life-threatening events due to tracheomalacia is aortopexy, either by thoracotomy or sternotomy. By lifting the aortic arch, the anterior wall of the trachea is lifted as well, increasing the diameter of the trachea. More recently, the aortopexy can also be carried out thoracoscopically.[14] Through a left-sided approach using a 5-mm trocar for the optic and two 3-mm trocars for instrumentation under endoscopic control, Ethibond 3-0 or 4-0 sutures can be brought in using a Reverdin needle to perforate the sternum, hooking up the adventitia of the aortic arch, and through the same stab incision pulled out again alongside the sternum with the use of an Endoclose needle retriever. Under direct flexible tracheoscopy through the endotracheal tube, the effect of lifting the aorta can be observed. The sutures are then tied subcutaneously onto the sternum.

More recently, the posterior tracheopexy against the prevertebral fascia has been described.[8,15] In this case, through a right thoracoscopy the esophagus is mobilized from the trachea in the same way an esophageal atresia would be approached. In case of an earlier esophageal atresia repair, the position of the esophagus is already in the right hemithorax. When the tracheomalacia is isolated, the position of the esophagus is more posterior and more in the way of the trachea to be fixed against the prevertebral fascia. But again, the esophagus has to be mobilized adequately for the pars membranacea to be attached to the prevertebral fascia with Ethibond 3-0 sutures. Usually 3 to 4 sutures are necessary. In more extensive cases, both an aortopexy and a posterior tracheopexy may be necessary. Depending on the condition of the child, this can be done in one single or in 2 separate procedures. When the tracheomalacia extends into the bronchi, aortopexy and/or tracheopexy will not suffice. There are some case reports whereby biodegradable 3-dimensional scaffolds have been used, tailored to the specific circumstances, that have been placed externally on the trachea and main bronchi as a splint with promising outcomes.

Reiterative Surgery

Recurrence of tracheoesophageal fistula in patients with esophageal atresia has been reported to occur in 5% to 10% of patients.[28,29] Depending on the circumstances, an attempt can be undertaken to close the fistula by cicatrization or with tissue glue.[30,31] If this fails, rethoracoscopy is necessary to close the fistula.[8] There usually is quite some scar tissue between the esophagus and trachea. Careful dissection is started inferiorly to come around the esophagus and introduce a vessel loop. Then the esophagus is mobilized cranially from the fistula and another vessel loop in introduced. With both vessel loops being pulled up, the fistula can now carefully be dissected under identification of the vagal branches. The tracheal side is closed with a transfixing suture. On the esophageal side, 2 stay sutures are placed in the corners before cutting the fistula. Thereafter the esophagus can be closed in a transverse fashion. There is no scientific evidence that interposition of tissue will preclude recurrence. A nasogastric tube is left behind for early feeding. Oral feeds may be started after 5 days. No contrast study is performed.

Recalcitrant Esophageal Stenosis

Esophageal stenosis is a frequently occurring complication after repair of esophageal atresia for which repetitive balloon dilatation may be necessary.[32] If the cicatrization is tight, dilatation with Savary dilators over a guidewire may be necessary. In the authors' department, they have developed a technique using the balloon dilator as an indwelling stent that is insufflated 3 times a day to let the esophagus heal in a predetermined diameter.[32] One of the reasons for recurrent stenosis may be gastro-esophageal reflux due to the pulling up of the distal esophagus, straightening the angle of His. If recurrent stenosis is persisting, a laparoscopic antireflux procedure may be indicated.[33] Nowadays partial fundoplication is preferred, as it causes less dysphagia, an issue that, particularly in patients with esophageal atresia, may hamper oral feeds. With the authors' management of an indwelling balloon catheter, they have been successful in solving recalcitrant stenoses, not only for esophageal atresia but also for extensive lye burns, for the last 12 years. Only recently for the first time the authors had to resect a stenosis that did not react to all of their conservative therapies. The approach was similar to the one used for congenital esophageal stenosis: mobilization of the esophagus. With the use of a balloon catheter in the esophagus or an esophagoscope, the exact level of the stenosis can be determined. The stenosis can be resected with an end-to-end anastomosis. A transanastomotic tube is introduced for early feeding. Principally no contrast study is performed, and oral feeds are started after 5 days. In another patient that was referred with a recurrent fistula and a persisting stenosis, the authors used the opportunity to close both the recurrent fistula and resect the stenosis in one thoracoscopic procedure.

Box 2
Follow-up protocol esophageal atresia

Follow-up

- Follow-up after 2, 4, and 8 weeks or earlier when indicated
  - Consultation with dietician (by telephone)
  - Consultation with pediatric pulmonologist (yearly, antibiotic prophylaxis during winter if necessary, lung function test at 6 years)
  - Consultation neonatologist (3, 6, 9, 12, 18, and 24 months with Bailey neurodevelopment tests)
  - Consultation pediatric gastroenterologist (esophagoscopy in case of stenosis or reflux; standard Barrett investigation at 12 and 17 years)
  - Consultation pediatrician
  - Consultation other specialists on indication
  - Regular follow-up at 3, 6, 9, and 12 months, then every 2 years thereafter

---

SUMMARY

Esophageal atresia is an anomaly with frequently occurring sequelae requiring lifelong management and follow-up (**Box 2**).

Because of the complex issues that may be encountered, patients with esophageal atresia preferably should be managed in centers of expertise that have the ability to deal with all types of anomalies and sequelae and can perform rigorous lifelong follow-up.

Tracheomalacia is an often-occurring concurrent anomaly that may cause acute life-threatening events and may warrant immediate management. In the past, major thoracotomies were necessary to carry out the artopexy. Nowadays aortpexy and posterior tracheopexy can both be performed thoracoscopically with quick recovery.

Best Practices

What is the current practice?

- Preoperative workup
- Preoperative rigid trachea-bronchoscopy
- Open or thoracoscopic correction of esophageal atresia

What changes in current practice are likely to improve outcomes?

- Multidisciplinary preoperative consultation on intended procedure
- Awareness of concomitant airway anomalies
- Life support course for parents
- Lifelong multidisciplinary follow-up

Clinical algorithm

Follow-up[1]
- Follow-up after 2, 4, and 8 weeks or earlier when indicated
  - Consultation with dietician (by telephone)
  - Consultation with pediatric pulmonologist (yearly, antibiotic prophylaxis during winter if necessary, lung function test at 6 years)
  - Consultation with neonatologist (3, 6, 9, 12, 18, and 24 months with Bailey neurodevelopment tests)
  - Consultation with pediatric gastroenterologist (esophagoscopy in case of stenosis or reflux; standard Barrett investigation at 12 and 17 years)

○ Consultation with pediatrician
○ Consultation with other specialists on indication
○ Regular follow-up with surgical team at 3, 6, 9, and 12 months, then every 2 years thereafter

Major recommendations

- Centralization into centers of expertise
- Development of quality standards for the management of esophageal atresia and upper airway pathology
- Lifelong follow-up with transition into adulthood
- Awareness of concomitant airway anomalies

Summary

Esophageal atresia is an anomaly with frequently occurring sequelae requiring lifelong management and follow-up. Because of the complex issues that can be encountered, patients with esophageal atresia preferably should be managed in centers of expertise that have the ability to deal with all types of anomalies and sequelae and can perform rigorous lifelong follow-up.

Tracheomalacia is an often-occurring concurrent anomaly that may cause acute life-threatening events and may warrant immediate management. In the past, major thoracotomies were necessary to carry out the aortopexy. Nowadays aortpexy and posterior tracheopexy can both be performed thoracoscopically with quick recovery.

REFERENCES

1. Krishnan U, Mousa H, Dall'Oglio L, et al. ESPGHAN-NASPGHAN guidelines for the evaluation and treatment of gastrointestinal and nutritional complications in children with esophageal atresia-tracheoesophageal fistula. J Pediatr Gastroenterol Nutr 2016;63(5):550–70.
2. Ludman L, Spitz L, Wade A. Educational attainments in early adolescence of infants who required major neonatal surgery. J Pediatr Surg 2001;36(6):858–62.
3. Block RI, Thomas JJ, Bayman EO, et al. Are anesthesia and surgery during infancy associated with altered academic performance during childhood? Anesthesiology 2012;117(3):494–503.
4. van Bel F, Lemmers P, Naulaers G. Monitoring neonatal regional cerebral oxygen saturation in clinical practice: value and pitfalls. Neonatology 2008;94(4):237–44.
5. Stolwijk LJ, Lemmers PM, Harmsen M, et al. Neurodevelopmental outcomes after neonatal surgery for major noncardiac anomalies [review]. Pediatrics 2016; 137(2):e20151728.
6. Stolwijk LJ, Keunen K, de Vries LS, et al. Neonatal surgery for noncardiac congenital anomalies: neonates at risk of brain injury. J Pediatr 2017;182:335–41.
7. Tytgat SH, van Herwaarden MY, Stolwijk LJ, et al. Neonatal brain oxygenation during thoracoscopic correction of esophageal atresia. Surg Endosc 2016;30(7): 2811–7.
8. Van der Zee DC. Semin Pediatr Surg 2017;26(2):67–71.
9. Bradshaw CJ, Thakkar H, Knutzen L, et al. Accuracy of prenatal detection of tracheoesophageal fistula and oesophageal atresia. J Pediatr Surg 2016;51(8): 1268–72.
10. Spaggiari E, Faure G, Rousseau V, et al. Performance of prenatal diagnosis in esophageal atresia. Prenat Diagn 2015;35(9):888–93.

11. Garabedian C, Sfeir R, Langlois C, et al. Does prenatal diagnosis modify neonatal management and early outcome of children with esophageal atresia type III? J Gynecol Obstet Biol Reprod (Paris) 2015;44(9):848–54 [in French].

12. Ethun CG, Fallon SC, Cassady CI, et al. Fetal MRI improves diagnostic accuracy in patients referred to a fetal center for suspected esophageal atresia. J Pediatr Surg 2014;49(5):712–5.

13. Hochart V, Verpillat P, Langlois C, et al. The contribution of fetal MR imaging to the assessment of oesophageal atresia. Eur Radiol 2015;25(2):306–14.

14. van der Zee DC, Straver M. Thoracoscopic aortopexy for tracheomalacia. World J Surg 2015;39(1):158–64.

15. Fraga JC, Jennings RW, Kim PC. Pediatric tracheomalacia. Semin Pediatr Surg 2016;25(3):156–64.

16. van der Zee DC, Tytgat SH, Zwaveling S, et al. Learning curve of thoracoscopic repair of esophageal atresia. World J Surg 2012;36(9):2093–7.

17. van der Zee DC, Gallo G, Tytgat SH. Thoracoscopic traction technique in long gap esophageal atresia: entering a new era. Surg Endosc 2015;29(11):3324–30.

18. van Poll D, van der Zee DC. Thoracoscopic treatment of congenital esophageal stenosis in combination with H-type tracheoesophageal fistula. J Pediatr Surg 2012;47(8):1611–3.

19. Bax KN, Roskott AM, van der Zee DC. Esophageal atresia without distal tracheoesophageal fistula: high incidence of proximal fistula. J Pediatr Surg 2008;43(3): 522–5.

20. van Der Zee DC, Bagolan P, Faure C, et al. Position paper of INoEA working group on long gap esophageal atresia: for better care. Front Pediatr 2017;5:63.

21. Lee HQ, Hawley A, Doak J, et al. Long-gap oesophageal atresia: comparison of delayed primary anastomosis and oesophageal replacement with gastric tube. J Pediatr Surg 2014;49(12):1762–6.

22. Long AM, Tyraskis A, Allin B, et al. Oesophageal atresia with no distal tracheoesophageal fistula: management and outcomes from a population-based cohort. J Pediatr Surg 2017;52(2):226–30.

23. Gallo G, Zwaveling S, Van der Zee DC, et al. A two-center comparative study of gastric pull-up and jejunal interposition for long gap esophageal atresia. J Pediatr Surg 2015;50(4):535–9.

24. Gallo G, Zwaveling S, Groen H, et al. Long-gap esophageal atresia: a meta-analysis of jejunal interposition, colon interposition, and gastric pull-up. Eur J Pediatr Surg 2012;22(6):420–5.

25. Bax NM, van der Zee DC. Jejunal pedicle grafts for reconstruction of the esophagus in children. J Pediatr Surg 2007;42(2):363–9.

26. Bairdain S, Foker JE, Smithers CJ, et al. Jejunal interposition after failed esophageal atresia repair. J Am Coll Surg 2016;222(6):1001–8.

27. Burgos L, Barrena S, Andrés AM, et al. Colonic interposition for esophageal replacement in children remains a good choice: 33-year median follow-up of 65 patients. J Pediatr Surg 2010;45(2):341–5.

28. Lal DR, Gadepalli SK, Downard CD, et al, Midwest Pediatric Surgery Consortium. Perioperative management and outcomes of esophageal atresia and tracheoesophageal fistula. J Pediatr Surg 2017;52(8):1245–51.

29. Smithers CJ, Hamilton TE, Manfredi MA, et al. Categorization and repair of recurrent and acquired tracheoesophageal fistulae occurring after esophageal atresia repair. J Pediatr Surg 2017;52(3):424–30.

30. Keckler SJ, St Peter SD, Calkins CM, et al. Occlusion of a recurrent tracheoesophageal fistula with surgisis. J Laparoendosc Adv Surg Tech A 2008;18(3):465–8.

31. Lelonge Y, Varlet F, Varela P, et al. Chemocauterization with trichloroacetic acid in congenital and recurrent tracheoesophageal fistula: a minimally invasive treatment. Surg Endosc 2016;30(4):1662–6.
32. van der Zee D, Hulsker C. Indwelling esophageal balloon catheter for benign esophageal stenosis in infants and children. Surg Endosc 2014;28(4):1126–30.
33. Mauritz FA, Conchillo JM, van Heurn LW, et al. Effects and efficacy of laparoscopic fundoplication in children with GERD: a prospective, multicenter study. Surg Endosc 2017;31(3):1101–10.

Minimally Invasive Patent Ductus Arteriosus Ligation

Alejandro V. Garcia, MD*, Jeffrey Lukish, MD

KEYWORDS

- Patent ductus arteriosus • Video-assisted thoracoscopic surgery
- Minimally invasive surgery • Premature infants • Surgical ligation • Neonate
- Congenital heart disease

KEY POINTS

- Patent ductus arteriosus is common, with an incidence of 1 to 2000, and represents 5% to 10% of all congenital heart anomalies.
- Persistent patent ductus arteriosus is associated with increased long-term morbidity and mortality related to the sequelae of a left-to-right shunt.
- Conservative management consists of mild fluid restriction, ventilator management, and prostaglandin inhibitor administration.
- Surgical ligation is reserved for infants with contraindications to medical management or who fail to improve with conservative measures.
- Both minimally invasive and open repairs have a high rate of success. The minimally invasive repair may provide improved exposure, shorter operative times, and a potential reduction in long-term morbidity from thoracogenic scoliosis.

Ligation of a patent ductus arteriosus (PDA) is a common procedure for infants who have hemodynamic sequela resulting from its patency and when closure cannot be achieved with medical therapy. The ligation of the PDA has continued to evolve since its first description in 1938 by Dr Robert Gross. With advancement in neonatal anesthesia and miniaturization of laparoscopic instruments, video-assisted thoracoscopic surgery (VATS) is now possible for even extremely low-birth-weight infants.[1] Thoracoscopic PDA ligation has been performed in infants as small as 500 g with good outcomes and low morbidity. Benefits of the thoracoscopic repair include decreased operative time, reduced postoperative pain, shorter hospital stay, and a potential for a reduction in the incidence of postoperative scoliosis.

The authors have no financial disclosures.
Department of Surgery, Division of Pediatric Surgery, Johns Hopkins University, 1800 Orleans Street, Bloomberg Building Suite 7310, Baltimore, MD 21287, USA
* Corresponding author.
E-mail address: Agarci41@jhmi.edu

Clin Perinatol 44 (2017) 763–771
http://dx.doi.org/10.1016/j.clp.2017.08.010
0095-5108/17/© 2017 Elsevier Inc. All rights reserved.

INTRODUCTION

A PDA is one of the most common congenital heart defects, representing 5% to 10% of all congenital heart cases.[2,3] A PDA results from the persistence of the fetal circulation with blood flow from the left pulmonary artery to the descending aorta. Its patency in utero is maintained by the high pulmonary vascular resistance by the nonaerated fluid-filled lungs. It remains patent due to a low circulating oxygen concentration and serum prostaglandins. After birth the lungs begin to aerate and receive increased blood flow. As the oxygen concentration increases and prostaglandins fall, the ductus begins to constrict. This constriction normally leads to intimal remodeling and closure, which typically occur within 72 hours of life for term newborns.[2,3] Lack of spontaneous closure leads to persistence of flow and shunt physiology and can be associated with significant morbidity and mortality.

EPIDEMIOLOGY

The incidence of a PDA in healthy term infants is 1 in 500 to 2000, which represents 5% to 10% of all congenital heart disease in term infants.[2–4] The risk of PDA is inversely proportional to birth weight and gestational age. The incidence in preterm infants less than 28 weeks of gestational age approaches 70% and in children 24 weeks' to 25 weeks' gestation the incidence is as high as 80%. Infants who are low birth weight are also at increased risk, with infants weighing less than 1200 g at birth having an incidence of 80%.[5]

In general, a ductus arteriosus spontaneously closes by 72 hours after birth. In infants greater than 30 weeks' gestation, 98% of PDAs close by the first week of life.[6] In infants under 24 weeks, the rate of spontaneous closure falls to 8% by day 4 and only 13% are closed by 1 week.[6] Early intervention may be required in severe cases due to hemodynamic instability and a high rate of morbidity and mortality. In those without significant sequela, a majority of defects are closed on reevaluation at 1 year of age.

PATHOPHYSIOLOGY

The clinical sequelae of a PDA are related to its size and flow dynamics with its subsequent effects on the heart. The higher left heart pressures result in an initial left-to-right shunt across the PDA. The size of the defect determines the degree of the shunt. A majority of early clinical morbidities are related to either pulmonary hyperperfusion or systemic hypoperfusion.[2,3,7] Hyperperfusion of the pulmonary vasculature results in pulmonary edema and may contribute to respiratory failure. Low systemic diastolic pressures may result in systemic hypoperfusion and acidosis, with an increased incidence of renal dysfunction, necrotizing enterocolitis (NEC), intraventricular hemorrhage (IVH) and prerenal azotemia.[2–4] A PDA is also associated with poor neurologic outcomes independent of IVH.[8]

In persistently patent moderate or large defects, increased work of the left ventricle may lead to hypertrophy and ultimately failure.[2,3] Persistently elevated pulmonary pressures due to long-standing pressure and volume overload can result in irreversible lung disease and pulmonary hypertension.[3,9,10] Increased workload of the right ventricle to overcome elevated pulmonary pressures can result in hypertrophy of the right ventricle.[3,9–11] In large PDAs, this may result in a reversal of flow in the ductus, with shunting of unoxygenated blood from the right ventricle into the systemic circulation, known as Eisenmenger syndrome.[9–11] Ultimately, persistent volume overload and increased work of the right ventricle may progress to right heart failure.[3,9–11]

With improved diagnostic capabilities and the availability of medical and invasive treatment, these sequelae are rarely seen in modern practice.

INITIAL EVALUATION

Most clinically significant PDAs are discovered in the neonatal period. Signs and symptoms are typically related to the size of the ductus. In the first 24 hours, neonates with clinically significant PDA typically have a decreased blood pressure due to delayed myocardial adaptation to changes in preload.[7] As the myocardium adapts, subsequent clinical signs may include bounding pulses, wide pulse pressures, and a characteristic machine-like murmur.[2,3,7] Clinically significant PDAs lead to signs of pulmonary overload on physical examination as well as respiratory distress, apneic episodes, and failure to wean from the ventilator. Diastolic hypotension and unexplained metabolic acidosis may also be observed.[2,3] These changes can lead to poor end organ perfusion and an increase in the incidence of NEC, renal failure, and IVH.[2–5] Presentation can range from poor feeding, failure to thrive, tachypnea, and diaphoresis to congestive heart failure in severe cases.

A diagnosis of a PDA is confirmed with an echocardiogram. This allows quantification of the severity of the defect and to rule out other ductal-dependent cardiac lesions that may be dependent on a PDA for systemic perfusion. Findings suggestive of a hemodynamically significant shunt include an absolute ductal diameter greater than 1.5 mm or a ratio of left atrial diameter to aortic diameter greater than or equal to 1.4, pulsatile low flow velocity in the descending aorta, or end-diastolic flow velocity in the left pulmonary artery greater than 0.20 m/s.[2–7] Chest radiographs may be used to evaluate the degree of pulmonary edema related to a clinically significant PDA.

MANAGEMENT

Given the lack of consensus as to what constitutes a clinically significant defect, a clear algorithm to guide management continues to be elusive. Given the increased risks associated with pharmacologic and surgical treatments, most recommendations favor a conservative approach for stable infants with minimal risk factors. Closure of asymptomatic PDAs is typically recommended by 2 years of age to minimize the risk of bacterial endocarditis and pulmonary hypertension.[5,6]

NONSURGICAL MANAGEMENT
Nonpharmacologic Management

For many infants without hemodynamic sequela of a PDA, nonpharmacologic management is considered appropriate. This involves a trial waiting period to allow for spontaneous closure. Conservative measures also include careful fluid management with mild fluid restriction and diuretics to avoid fluid overload and prevent lung injury while maintaining adequate end organ perfusion.[2,5–7] Increasing pulmonary vascular resistance by lowering inspiratory time and increasing positive end-expiratory pressure may encourage closure for infants who are ventilator dependent.[6,7]

Pharmacologic Management

Prostaglandin inhibitors remain the cornerstone of medical therapy for remodeling and closure of a PDA.[2,3,5–7] Typically, nonsteroidal anti-inflammatory drugs, such as intravenous indomethacin, are used. Early studies advocated for early prophylactic use of prostaglandin inhibitors to minimize the incidence of complications related to a PDA.[5,6] Further studies demonstrated, however, potential pulmonary morbidity from a possible increased frequency of bronchopulmonary dysplasia within the first year of life. Prostaglandin inhibitors may also have detrimental effects on the mesenteric, cerebral, and renal circulation, limiting its widespread use. Current recommendations suggest the use of prostaglandin inhibitors as initial therapy for hemodynamically significant defects as suggested by symptoms or electrocardiogram.[5–7]

Transarterial Occlusion

Transarterial occlusion via endovascular techniques is the standard approach for PDA closure in adults and term infants who have failed medical therapy. Recent evidence has suggested that this technique may also be used safely in smaller infants.[12,13] Studies have demonstrated that transarterial closure can be highly successful with low rates of complications even in preterm and very low-birth-weight infants.[5,6,12,13] Long-term studies are needed to determine the long-term viability of this approach for infants.

SURGICAL MANAGEMENT

Review of the literature reveals no significant difference between medical and surgical intervention with regard to success rates or mortality. The timing of intervention and indications for surgical ligation are highly debated in the literature. In general, surgical ligation is indicated for infants who fail to stabilize after medical management.[2,5,7,14–16] Surgical ligation has been shown to facilitate extubation in infants with left ventricular overload and decrease the risk of consequences from systemic hypoperfusion.[5,6,16] Premature infants with hemodynamically significant defects may benefit from surgical closure because they are less likely to respond to medical therapy and they tend not to tolerate instability from prolonged nonsurgical treatment. Early surgical ligation should also be considered with clinical significant defects in which medical treatment is contraindicated. Nonsteroidal anti-inflammatory drugs are typically avoided in infants with NEC, acute renal failure, IVH, or other evidence of bleeding in the pulmonary or gastrointestinal tract.[5–7,14–17]

Surgical Approach

Both open and thoracoscopic approaches to PDA repair are well tolerated, with low rates of morbidity and mortality.[14–24] The thoracoscopic repair was first described by Laborde and colleagues[21] in 1993. This approach has become the standard approach at many centers.[17–19,21–24] Recent reports demonstrate that this technique can be safely applied to very low-birth-weight and extremely low-birth-weight infants.[22–24] Minimally invasive approaches have the potential advantage of improved visualization to minimize risk of injury to surrounding structures. Studies have shown that the thoracoscopic approach is associated with decreased operative time, smaller incisions with less postoperative pain, earlier extubation, and decreased hospital and ICU stay compared with the open approach.[17–19] The thoracoscopic approach also avoids potential long-term scoliosis due to avoidance of rib spreading, muscular division, nerve injury, and rupture of intercostal ligaments.[17–19] Proponents of the open technique point out that vascular control in cases of hemorrhage may be more challenging using the thoracoscopic approach. Those cases in which conversion from thoracoscopy to open repair is required can be safely completed with a standard thoracotomy with no added morbidity.[25,26]

Minimally Invasive Thoracoscopic Repair Technique

After induction of general anesthesia, the infant is placed in the right lateral decubitus position. Three incisions are placed along the fifth intercostal space at the site of an intended thoracotomy incision should an open procedure become necessary. The initial 3-mm incision is made in the left fifth intercostal space in the posterior axillary line. After placement of a 3-mm port, thoracoscopy is performed. During this phase of the operation, low-volume carbon dioxide insufflation is used with a pressure set at 6 mm of mercury and flow rate of 0.5 L/min. A second 3-mm incision is made in the left fifth intercostal space in the midaxillary line (**Fig. 1**). Via this site, a 3-mm fan retractor (Karl Storz GmbH and Company, Munich, Germany) that was previously modified using a plastic towel drape (Medical Concepts Development, St. Paul, Minnesota) is inserted without a port under direct visualization (**Fig. 2**). Once the fan retractor is used to retract the lung, insufflation is discontinued. With gentle retraction of the right midlung and apical lung, the aortic arch, descending aorta, left subclavian artery, and PDA should be clearly visualized (**Fig. 3**). The recurrent laryngeal nerve should be identified as it crosses over the medial aspect of the ductus. A final 5-mm incision is made posteriorly in the fifth intercostal space approximately 1 cm below the inferior tip of the scapula. A 3-mm curved dissector is used to begin dissection medial to the descending aorta just below the presumptive PDA/aortic junction. The junction is further defined by the dissection of the PDA inferiorly and superiorly. Care should be taken to avoid unnecessary traction on the recurrent laryngeal nerve. Gentle dissection continues along the superior and inferior edges of the PDA, freeing it from surrounding tissue and carefully defining the ductus until it has been exposed nearly circumferentially. Dissection proceeds toward the pulmonary artery until a small segment is clearly defined for optimal placement of 2 clips. It is the practice of the

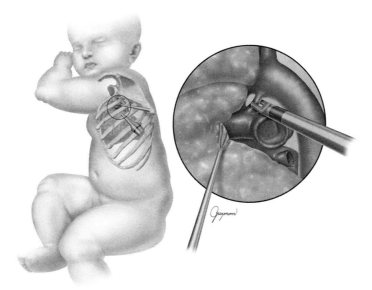

Fig. 1. A 3-mm port is placed in the left fifth intercostal space in the posterior axillary line. A second 3-mm incision is made in the left fifth intercostal space in the midaxillary line. Via this site, a 3-mm fan retractor is inserted without a port under direct visualization. Once the fan retractor is used to retract the lung, insufflation is discontinued. A final 5-mm incision is made posteriorly in the fifth intercostal space approximately 1 cm below the inferior tip of the scapula. This port is used for a curved dissector for dissection and a clip applier for ligation of PDA.

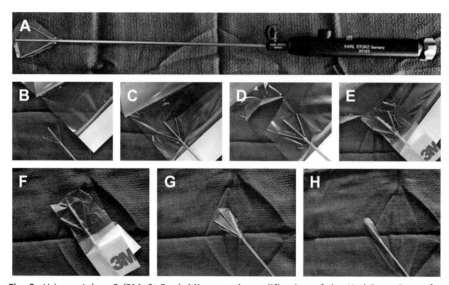

Fig. 2. Using a Ioban 2 (3M, St Paul, Minnesota), modification of the Karl Storz 3-mm fan retractor is constructed as follows. (*A*) Modified fan retractor. (*B*) Ioban drape is opened in the sterile field. (*C*) Open fan retractor is placed open approximately 2 cm from end of Ioban drape. (*D*) The Ioban drape is cut one inch above the end of the drape. (*E*) The instrument is rotated 180° to cover the instrument 360°. (*F*) The Ioban drape is cut one inch off the open side. (*G*) The ends of the Ioban drape are folded around the open instrument. (*H*) The instrument is ready to be used and can be closed for introduction into the thorax.

authors to perform a test occlusion prior to clipping the duct while monitoring preductal and postductal oxygen saturations as well as observing the lung to look for any changes in perfusion.

After test occlusion, the clip applier (Weck Horizon, Teleflex, Limerick, Pennsylvania) is inserted through the posterior 5-mm working port and 2 medium metal clips

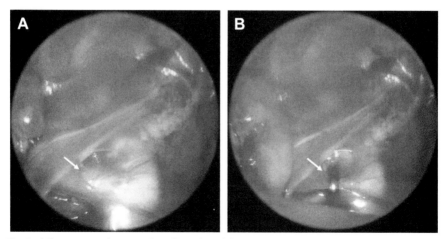

Fig. 3. (*A*) Arrow marks PDA after dissection. (*B*) Arrow marks 2 medium metal clips applied near the PDA junction with the aorta.

are applied near the PDA junction with the aorta. The area is inspected for optimal clip placement and hemostasis and the thoracic cavity is examined once again to rule out any evidence of lung injury. The incisions are then closed in the standard fashion. Prior to closure of the last incision, positive inspiratory pressure is applied to fully inflate the lung to facilitate evacuation of the pneumothorax. The authors do not routinely place thoracostomy tubes in the absence of suspected lung injury.

At the authors' institution, 31 premature infants underwent VATS PDA ligation. Mean weight of the infants at the time of operation was 810 g (range 580–1150 g). The operative times ranged from 18 to 35 minutes; 29 of the procedures were completed successfully thoracoscopically. Two children were converted to thoracotomy due to instability. One of these children represent the only postoperative death within 72 hours of the procedure in the study group. Five other infants died during hospitalization from etiologies unrelated to the PDA ligation. All 29 infants had documented successful ligation by postoperative echocardiogram. One infant had prolonged intubation from a recurrent laryngeal nerve injury. Six-month postoperative bronchoscopy in this infant revealed normal vocal cord movement.

POSTOPERATIVE MANAGEMENT

After surgical repair, a chest radiograph should be performed to rule out pneumothorax and an echocardiogram performed to confirm occlusion of flow across the PDA.[22–25] Abrupt hemodynamic changes may occur after surgical ligation. Typically, there is an increase in diastolic arterial pressure and an associated increase in the mean arterial pressure.[17] In the immediate postoperative period, however, this increase in mean arterial pressure often fails to reach normal levels. This may lead to a transient decrease in postoperative cerebral perfusion and an increase in the oxygenation index after ligation.[17] These hemodynamic changes require careful titration of fluids and vasopressors to maintain adequate perfusion while avoiding pulmonary edema.

COMPLICATIONS

Mortality after thoracoscopic repair of a PDA is reported to be less than 1%. Intraoperative hemorrhage is also uncommon with reported rates between 0.5% and 1%.[18–21,23–25] Major vascular injuries to the pulmonary artery and descending aorta are exceedingly rare.[27,28] Morbidity after PDA ligation typically involves injury to the recurrent laryngeal nerve with a reported range of 0.5% to 6%. Rates of pneumothorax are between 0.5% to 6% and rates of chylothorax are noted to be between 0.5% to 3%. No significant differences were seen between the open and thoracoscopic approaches in regard to recurrent laryngeal nerve injuries, pneumothorax or chylothorax.[18–20,22,24] Greater than half of injuries to the recurrent laryngeal nerve are transient and spontaneous full return of function is often noted.[19–21] Postoperative mortality approaches 15% in some reports, with the highest incidence in premature and low-birth-weight infants.[15,19,24] The most common cause of in-hospital death was sepsis commonly associated with NEC. Chronic lung disease and multisystem organ failure are also commonly seen in these infants.[15,19,24]

SUMMARY

The minimally invasive repair of a PDA is a safe and effective procedure even in premature and low-birth-weight infants. This approach offers many advantages over the open approach with less postoperative pain, earlier extubation, and shorter hospital and ICU stays. Thoracoscopy also allows improved visualization and shorter operative times and a potential reduction in thoracogenic scoliosis.

Best Practices

What is the current practice?

- The traditional management for a PDA that has been refractory to medical management has been via a thoracotomy to allow ligation.
- A possible sequela to a thoracotomy is the risk of long-term musculoskeletal changes that may lead to scoliosis.

What changes in current practice are likely to improve outcomes?

- Newer thoracoscopic procedures are feasible even in small premature infants and may avoid long-term morbidity.
- Thoracoscopic approaches have been associated with a very low rate of complications or morbidity compared with the open technique
- Newer instruments have been designed to allow adequate exposure during minimally invasive approaches in infants

Major recommendations

- Thoracoscopic approaches should be considered to ligate a PDA to avoid the long-term sequelae of a thoracotomy on chest wall development.

ACKNOWLEDGMENTS

Special thanks to William Guzman, Jr for his assistance with the artwork for this article.

REFERENCES

1. Lukish J. Video-assisted thoracoscopic ligation of a patent ductus arteriosus in a very low-birth-weight infant using a novel retractor. J Pediatr Surg 2009;44: 1047–50.
2. Dice J, Bhatia J. Patent ductus arteriosus: an overview. J Pediatr Pharmacol Ther 2007;12:138–46.
3. Schneider D. The patent ductus arteriosus in term infants, children, and adults. Semin Perinatol 2011;36:146–53.
4. Lloyd TR, Beekman RH III. Clinically silent patent ductus arteriosus [Letter]. Am Heart J 1994;127:1664–5.
5. Heuchan AM, Clyman RI. Managing the patent ductus arteriosus: current treatment options. Arch Dis Child Fetal Neonatal Ed 2014;99:431–6.
6. Mitra S, Ronnestad A, Holmstrom H. Management of patent ductus arteriosus in preterm infants- where do we stand? Congenit Heart Dis 2013;8:500–12.
7. Jain A, Shah P. Diagnosis, evaluation, and management of patent ductus arteriosus in preterm neonates. JAMA Pediatr 2015;169(9):863–72.
8. Weisz DE, McNamara PJ. Patent ductus arteriosus ligation and adverse outcomes: causality or bias? J Clin Neonatol 2014;3(2):67–75.
9. Kriege EV, Learly PJ, Opotowsky AR. Pulmonary hypertension in congenital heart disease: beyond Eisenmenger syndrome. Cardiol Clin 2015;33(4):599–609.
10. Schneider DJ, Moore JQ. Congenital heart disease for the adult cardiologist. Circulation 2006;114:1873–82.

11. Waddell TK, Bennett L, Kennedy R, et al. Heart-lung or lung transplantation for Eisenmenger syndrome. J Heart Lung Transplant 2002;21:731–7.

12. Francis E, Singhi AK, Lakshmivenkateshaiah S, et al. Transcatheter occlusion of patent ductus arteriosus in pre-term infants. JACC Cardiovasc Interv 2010;3(5): 550–5.

13. Baruteau AE, Hascoet S, Baruteau J, et al. Transcatheter closure of patent ductus arteriosus: past present and future. Arch Cardiovasc Dis 2014;107(2):122–32.

14. Weinberg JG, Evans FJ, Burns KM, et al. Surgical ligation of patent ductus arteriosus in premature infants: trends and practice variation. Cardiol Young 2016; 26(6):1107–14.

15. Lee LC, Tillett A, Tulloh R, et al. Outcome following patent ductus arteriosus ligation in premature infants: a retrospective cohort analysis. BMC Pediatr 2006;6:15.

16. Tashiro J, Perez EA, Sola JE. Reduced hospital mortality with surgical ligation of patent ductus arteriosus in premature, extremely low birth weight infants: a propensity score-matched outcome study. Ann Surg 2016;263(3):608–14.

17. Teixeria LS, Shivananda SP, Stephens D, et al. Postoperative cardiorespiratory instability following ligation of the preterm ductus arteriosus is related to early need for intervention. J Perinatol 2008;28:803–10.

18. Chen H, Weng G, Chen Z, et al. Comparison of posterolateral thoracotomy and video-assisted thoracoscopic clipping for the treatment of patent ductus arteriosus in neonates and infants. Pediatr Cardiol 2011;32:386–90.

19. Stankowski T, Aboul-Hassan SS, Marczak J, et al. Is thoracoscopic patent ductus arteriosus closure superior to conventional surgery? Interact Cardiovasc Thorac Surg 2015;21:532–8.

20. Vanamo K, Berg E, Kokki H, et al. Video-assisted thoracoscopic versus open surgery for persistent ductus arteriosus. J Pediatr Surg 2006;41:1226–9.

21. Laborde F, Noirhomme R, Karam J, et al. A new video-assisted thoracoscopic surgical technique for interruption of patent ductus arteriosus in infants and children. J Thorac Cardiovasc Surg 1993;105:278–80.

22. Nezafati MH, Soltani G, Vedadian A. Video-assisted ductal closure with new modifications: minimally invasive, maximally effective, 1300 cases. Ann Thorac Surg 2007;84:1343–8.

23. Slater B, Rothenberg S. Thoracoscopic management of patent ductus arteriosus and vascular rings in infants and children. J Laparoendosc Adv Surg Tech 2015; 25:1–4.

24. Hines MH, Raines KH, Payne RM. Video-assisted ductal ligation in premature infants. Ann Thorac Surg 2003;76:1417–20.

25. Stankowski T, Aboul-Hassan SS, Marczak J, et al. Minimally invasive thoracoscopic closure versus thoracotomy in children with patent ductus arteriosis. J Surg Res 2017;208:1–9.

26. Fuller SJ, Gruber PJ. Patent ductus arteriosus. In: Mattei P, editor. Fundamentals of pediatric surgery. New York: Springer-Verlag; 2011. p. 283–8.

27. Grunenfelder J, Bartram U, Van Praagh R, et al. The large window ductus: a surgical trap. Ann Thorac Surg 1998;65(6):1790–1.

28. Tefera E, Bermudez-Canete R, van Doorn C. Inadvertent ligation of the left pulmonary artery during intended ductal ligation. BMC Res Notes 2015;8:511.

Congenital Diaphragmatic Hernia and Diaphragmatic Eventration

Matthew S. Clifton, MD, Mark L. Wulkan, MD*

KEYWORDS

- Congenital diaphragmatic hernia • CDH • Morgagni hernia • Bochdalek hernia

KEY POINTS

- Congenital diaphragmatic hernia (CDH) occurs in approximately 1 in 2500 to 5000 children.
- The lack of uniform early diagnosis and referral has led to discrepancies in reporting incidence and survival, and resulted in the "hidden mortality."
- Two main types of CDH occur: Morgagni (anteromedial) and Bochdalek (posterolateral).
- Bochdalek hernias occur at a much greater frequency, and are typically associated with physiologic derangements in the newborn.

INTRODUCTION: NATURE OF THE PROBLEM

Congenital diaphragmatic hernia (CDH) occurs in approximately 1 in 2500 to 5000 children. The lack of uniform early diagnosis and referral has led to discrepancies in reporting incidence and survival, and resulted in "hidden mortality," a term coined by Dr Michael Harrison in 1978. Two main types of CDH occur: Morgagni (anteromedial) and Bochdalek (posterolateral). Because Bochdalek hernias occur with much higher frequency, and are typically associated with physiologic derangements in the newborn, they are the focus of this article. Repair of the hernia can take many forms, with an open or minimally invasive technique, with or without a patch, and approached from the abdomen or thorax. The attendant pulmonary hypertension and hypoplasia experienced by patients with CDH are the main determinants of survival, and therefore the focus of perinatal management.

INDICATIONS AND CONTRAINDICATIONS

Congenital anomalies of the diaphragm span the range of disease severity, from an asymptomatic mild eventration resulting from shoulder dystocia during childbirth to

Department of Surgery, Division of Pediatric Surgery, Emory University School of Medicine, 1405 Clifton Road NE, Atlanta, GA 30322, USA
* Corresponding author.
E-mail address: mwulkan@emory.edu

Clin Perinatol 44 (2017) 773–779
http://dx.doi.org/10.1016/j.clp.2017.08.011   perinatology.theclinics.com
0095-5108/17/© 2017 Elsevier Inc. All rights reserved.

complete absence of the diaphragm in the setting of a severe Bochdalek hernia. The indication for surgery in diaphragmatic hernia patients is straightforward—the presence of a hernia necessitates repair almost universally. The exception to this is an infant who is so profoundly unstable with no chance of recovery or adaptation of the pulmonary pressures.

SURGICAL TECHNIQUE AND PROCEDURE
Preoperative Planning

Management of the patient with CDH before surgery can take several different forms in terms of repair timing, but all hold several basic tenets in place: permissive hypercapnia (target range of $Paco_2$, 45–60 mm Hg), maintenance of preductal oxygen saturation (goal of 85%–95%), minimize volutrauma and barotrauma with conventional ventilator strategies aimed at keeping a positive inspiratory pressure of less than 25 cm H_2O with a positive end-expiratory pressure of between 2 and 5 cm H_2O. If this cannot be accomplished, conversion to high-frequency oscillatory ventilation is used, optimizing alveolar recruitment with a mean arterial pressure of 13 to 17.[1–3] The addition of inhaled nitric oxide can further decompress the pulmonary vascular bed. Pressors may be necessary, aimed at driving up inotropy. If these goals cannot be accomplished using maximal medical therapy, extracorporeal membrane oxygenation (ECMO) is required to deliver oxygen and remove CO_2. The typical indication for ECMO is a sustained oxygen index of greater than 35 to 40. At our institution, we typically await resolution of increased pulmonary artery pressures before proceeding with repair. These signs include decreased pulmonary artery pressures (using preductal arterial oxygen saturation as a surrogate marker, indicating a low degree of right-to-left shunting), along with decreased pressor requirement, and echocardiography showing decreased signs of right ventricular strain.[4] Use of ECMO beyond 4 weeks duration has been disputed.[5] At other institutions, the CDH is repaired early while still on ECMO.[6] Blood products are prepared in advance for the almost certain need for perioperative transfusion.

Preparation and Patient Positioning

The infant is laid across the operating table at the end of the bed such that the face is directed toward the anesthesiologist. The patient is placed in the lateral decubitus position with the affected side up, and the body prepped from the shoulder to the pelvis, including the abdomen. The head is placed at a slightly obtuse angle leaning toward the unaffected side, beyond midline, so as to minimize instrument strike while working thoracoscopically. An axillary roll is placed to protect the brachial plexus (depending on patient size, this may be a gel roll or soft gauze), and the patient is secured to the bed. An additional roll is placed to support the back. The surgeon and assistant stand at the head of the bed and a screen is positioned near the patient's feet. In the event that conversion to an open procedure is necessary, the tape securing the baby is split by a nurse, maintaining sterility, and the roll removed from behind the back.

Surgical Approach

These authors prefer a thoracoscopic approach for both CDH and eventration, regardless of the side. This allows for a better suturing angle and facilitates reduction of the viscera in a CDH.[7] We use the thoracoscopic approach for any infant that is stable enough to be transported to the operating room. If the infant is requiring high ventilator support or is on ECMO, and hence too unstable to be transported, we perform an open repair in the neonatal intensive care unit.

Surgical Procedure: Congenital Diaphragmatic Hernia

Step one: establish safe access to the chest
During thoracoscopy, the initial entry point is anterior to the tip of the scapula at the fourth intercostal space. Two additional ports are placed, one at the anterior and one at the posterior axillary line. An additional trocar can be placed to assist with retraction or visceral manipulation; however, it is usually not necessary. If conversion to an open operation is necessary, a subcostal incision is made and extended laterally. With the affected side slightly tilted up, access to the diaphragm is improved (**Fig. 1**).

Step two: reduce the abdominal viscera beneath the diaphragm
This step requires an awareness of the positioning of the patient. The open area in the peritoneal space is slightly anterior, not directly ahead, when reducing the viscera. This prevents injury to the intestine and the retroperitoneal structures. On left sided defects, the spleen is typically used as a "cap" to keep the hollow viscera at bay. Once the viscera are reduced, the insufflation pressure can be reduced or even stopped to facilitate a more "normal" diaphragm position during closure and to help minimize the $Paco_2$.

Step three: assess the size of the defect relative to the surface area of the affected hemidiaphragm
A small defect can be closed primarily, whereas a larger defect requires a prosthetic patch (**Fig. 2**).

Step four: unfurl the trapped diaphragm
Often there is additional diaphragmatic muscle that can be used in closure.

Step five: formal defect closure with either open or thoracoscopic approach
A primary repair is reinforced using 6-ply SIS (a bioprosthetic mesh) placed on the abdominal side of the defect.[8] Descriptions of thoracoscopic closure vary, with some authors moving lateral to medial, others medial to lateral.[9] The bioprosthetic mesh is incorporated in the interrupted suture line. The authors prefer to use silk suture. To approximate the muscle at the furthest lateral recess of the costophrenic angle, a triangular stitch is taken, passing the needle through a stab wound in the skin, down through the intercostal space, through both leaflets of diaphragm, then back up through the skin incision, passing the needle on the opposite site of the

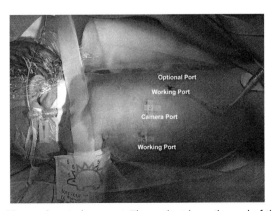

Fig. 1. Patient position and port placement. The patient is on the end of the table sideways. The surgeon stands at the patient's head.

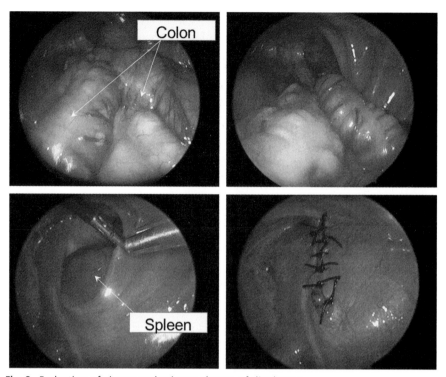

Fig. 2. Reduction of viscera and primary closure of diaphragm.

nearest rib (the so-called pericostal stitch).[10] Thoracoscopic repair is ideal for defects that can be addressed with primary closure. Use of a small Gore-tex (W.L. Gore & Associates, Flagstaff, AZ) patch laterally in the absence of adequate muscle is reasonable, but the quality of the repair should never be compromised in an effort to maintain a minimally invasive approach.[11] Close attention should be paid to the patient's $Paco_2$ during the operation—a lengthy operation should be avoided. As such, a skilled technician capable of intracorporeal knot tying is critical to a safe, successful closure performed thoracoscopically.

Larger defects requiring a patch are best repaired in an open fashion, using a Gore-tex patch sewn directly to the diaphragm in an interrupted, horizontal mattress fashion. The Gore-tex patch is cut to be 1 cm larger than the defect circumferentially. The posterior row is placed first, parachuting the sutures all down at once. This should produce a "dome" effect on the neodiaphragm. A bioprosthetic patch cut 2 cm larger circumferentially relative to the size of the defect is placed on the abdominal side of the diaphragm. This patch is tacked in several places to prevent the patch from being displaced (**Figs. 3** and **4**).

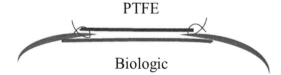

Fig. 3. Polytetrafluoroethylene (PTFE) is used to bridge the gap with a larger biologic underlay.

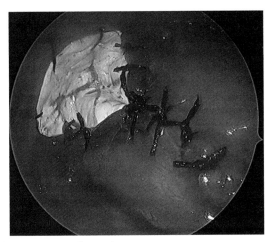

Fig. 4. Completed composite mesh repair.

A decision to place a chest tube or not depends on the surgeon's preference.[1,2,12] Even a small amount of air leak from the affected lung can cause substantial mediastinal shift. It is known that the obligate pneumothorax will be replaced by a hydrothorax in the days after surgery. Concerns regarding infection of the prosthetic patch have been unfounded to date.

COMPLICATIONS AND THEIR MANAGEMENT

Complications stemming from repair of CDH are best divided into early and late. As mentioned, early pneumothorax or hydrothorax can necessitate a tube thoracostomy.[12] This procedure centralizes the mediastinum, improves venous return to the heart, and maintains systemic perfusion. Occasionally, an abdominal compartment syndrome can result from lack of abdominal domain and the rapid replacement of the viscera in a contained space. In this setting, ideal management is decompressive laparotomy, with skin flaps raised for closure to keep the intestine covered with a biological dressing.

The most notable late complication is recurrent hernia. Signs of recurrence can include dyspnea, tachypnea, and poor feeding; however, some recurrences are occult and present only on screening chest radiograph. Recurrences can be approached with laparoscopy, thoracoscopy, laparotomy, thoracotomy, or a hybrid approach.[13] A key to management of recurrence is to provide a tension-free repair—often this means the use of a prosthetic mesh to bridge the gap in muscle coverage. Patients who have undergone open repair of a CDH are at a significantly increased risk of small bowel obstruction. Review of our institutional data of 144 patients over the past 10 years showed a statistically significant increase in the incidence of bowel obstruction in patients undergoing open repair of CDH (14.3% in patients repaired open, 0% in patients reported thoracoscopically, unpublished data, Bhatia AM and Wulkan ML, 2016). These results were consistent irrespective of the use of a primary repair or patch repair. Management is the same as with any bowel obstruction—patients with a complete obstruction or peritonitis warrant immediate operation; those with partial obstructions and a benign examination can be observed, keeping a low threshold to move forward with an operation if their condition deteriorates. An additional long-term postoperative consideration for CDH patients is skeletal deformity, which can take the form of abnormal spinal curvature and chest wall asymmetry. This requires close follow-up with a multidisciplinary clinic or spine surgeon.[14,15] Gastroesophageal reflux disease is quite common in CDH patients, and is typically managed medically.[15] Occasionally, an antireflux operation is warranted to prevent reflux related lung soilage.

POSTOPERATIVE CARE

Early postoperative care of patients with CDH is supportive and aimed at weaning the ventilator and managing the pulmonary hypertension. Feeding is initiated with careful attention paid to gastroesophageal reflux disease–related problems. Once home, patients are followed every 3 months as an outpatient for the first year with concurrent chest radiographs to assess for recurrence. The majority of recurrences happen during the first 12 months after repair, likely related to the dramatic growth experienced by infants in the first year of life. For the second year postoperatively, visits are spaced out to every 6 months, again with chest radiographs. Thereafter, patients are seen on an annual basis with concurrent chest radiographs.

OUTCOMES

The main outcome studied for CDH repair is recurrence. In our dataset, there was a trend toward a higher recurrence rate in patients repaired using a minimally invasive approach, though it did not reach statistical significance (3.9% vs 7.8% for primary repairs, and 24% vs 33% for patch repairs). Bowel obstructions, as referenced, remain a source of morbidity for patients undergoing an open repair, regardless of the use of a Gore-tex or bioprosthetic patch. After risk stratification by defect size and patient characteristics, the trend toward increased recurrence in minimally invasive repairs and increased rates of small bowel obstruction in open repairs has been validated by the CDH Study Group.[16] Chylothorax can occur, although it is relatively uncommon (3.9% of primary repairs, and 6.9% of patch repairs). Developmental delay, musculoskeletal deformity, hearing impairment, and gastroesophageal reflux disease are common morbidities. A recent study of a cohort of CDH patients led by Dr. Holly Hedrick[17] found that the rates of borderline or extremely low IQ were increased in CDH patients when compared with their healthy counterparts. Owing to the number and complexity of long-term morbidities, a multidisciplinary clinic is frequently used to streamline management.

SUMMARY

CDH can be approached successfully using minimally invasive techniques. Although there are may be a suggestion of higher recurrence rates with thoracoscopic repair, this may be due to the learning curve. In addition, you trade off a higher rate of small bowel obstruction with open repair. Appropriate patients who have CDH should be offered the benefits of minimally invasive repair.

REFERENCES

1. Boloker J, Bateman DA, Wung JT, et al. Congenital diaphragmatic hernia in 120 infants treated consecutively with permissive hypercapnea/spontaneous respiration/elective repair. J Pediatr Surg 2002;37(3):357–66.
2. Wung JT, Sahni R, Moffitt ST, et al. Congenital diaphragmatic hernia: survival treated with very delayed surgery, spontaneous respiration, and no chest tube. J Pediatr Surg 1995;30(3):406–9.

3. Tracy ET, Mears SE, Smith PB, et al. Protocolized approach to the management of congenital diaphragmatic hernia: benefits of reducing variability in care. J Pediatr Surg 2010;45(6):1343–8.
4. Geggel RL, Murphy JD, Langleben D, et al. Congenital diaphragmatic hernia: arterial structural changes and persistent pulmonary hypertension after surgical repair. J Pediatr 1985;107(3):457–64.
5. Kays DW, Islam S, Richards DS, et al. Extracorporeal life-support of patients with congenital diaphragmatic hernia: how long should we treat? J Am Coll Surg 2014; 218(4):808–17.
6. Hollinger LE, Lally PA, Tsao K, et al, Congenital Diaphragmatic Hernia Study Group. A risk-stratified analysis of delayed congenital diaphragmatic hernia repair: does timing of operation matter? Surgery 2014;156(2):475–82.
7. Holcomb GW 3rd, Georgeson KE, Rothenberg SE. Atlas of pediatric laparoscopy and thoracoscopy. Philadelphia: Saunders Elsevier; 2008.
8. Gonzalez R, Hill SJ, Mattar SG, et al. Absorbable versus nonabsorbable mesh repair of congenital diaphragmatic hernias in a growing animal model. J Laparoendosc Adv Surg Tech A 2011;21(5):449–54.
9. Shah SR, Wishnew J, Barsness K, et al. Minimally invasive congenital diaphragmatic hernia repair: a 7-year review of one institution's experience. Surg Endosc 2009;23(6):1265–71.
10. Rozmiarek A, Weinsheimer R, Azzie G. Primary thoracoscopic repair of diaphragmatic hernia with pericostal sutures. J Laparoendosc Adv Surg Tech A 2005; 15(6):667–9.
11. Keijzer R, van de Ven C, Vlot J, et al. Thoracoscopic repair in congenital diaphragmatic hernia: patching is safe and reduces the recurrence rate. J Pediatr Surg 2010;45(5):953–7.
12. Schlager A, Arps K, Siddharthan R, et al. Tube thoracostomy at the time of congenital diaphragmatic hernia repair: reassessing the risks and benefits. J Laparoendosc Adv Surg Tech A 2017;27(3):311–7.
13. Bruns NE, Glenn IC, McNinch NL, et al. Approach to recurrent congenital diaphragmatic hernia: results of an international survey. J Laparoendosc Adv Surg Tech A 2016;26(11):925–9.
14. Jancelewicz T, Vu LT, Keller RL, et al. Long-term surgical outcomes in congenital diaphragmatic hernia: observations from a single institution. J Pediatr Surg 2010; 45(1):155–60 [discussion:60].
15. Nobuhara KK, Lund DP, Mitchell J, et al. Long-term outlook for survivors of congenital diaphragmatic hernia. Clin Perinatol 1996;23(4):873–87.
16. Putnam LR, Tsao K, Lally KP, et al. Minimally invasive vs open congenital diaphragmatic hernia repair: is there a superior approach? J Am Coll Surg 2017; 224(4):416–22.
17. Danzer E, Hoffman C, D'Agostino JA, et al. Neurodevelopmental outcomes at 5years of age in congenital diaphragmatic hernia. J Pediatr Surg 2017;52(3): 437–43.

Thoracoscopic Lobectomy for Congenital Lung Lesions

Jarrett Moyer, MD[a],*, Hanmin Lee, MD[b], Lan Vu, MD[b]

KEYWORDS

- Congenital • Lung • Lesion • Malformation • Thoracoscopic • Resection
- Lobectomy • CPAM

KEY POINTS

- Most congenital lung lesions are diagnosed on prenatal ultrasound.
- Most fetuses with congenital lung lesions proceed to uncomplicated term delivery.
- Thoracoscopic lobectomy is safe, well-tolerated, and results in a shorter length of hospital stay compared with open resection.
- Symptomatic neonates should undergo resection shortly after birth.
- Asymptomatic neonates can be observed and undergo prophylactic resection at 6 months of life or later.

INTRODUCTION

Congenital lung lesions (CLLs) comprise a heterogeneous collection of rare developmental parenchymal lung abnormalities present in utero and at birth, including congenital pulmonary airway malformation (CPAM), bronchopulmonary sequestration (intralobar and extralobar), bronchial atresia, and congenital lobar emphysema. Additionally, pleuropulmonary blastoma (PPB), mediastinal teratoma, and bronchogenic cysts can mimic CLLs on fetal ultrasonography, postnatal radiograph, and postnatal contrast-enhanced computed tomography (CT) or MRI. CLLs are often diagnosed on prenatal ultrasound and have overlapping radiologic features. Thus, definitive diagnosis relies on histopathologic analysis of resected tissue.[1] Given the heterogeneity of CLL, it is not surprising that these lesions carry unpredictable and vastly different clinical outcomes if left untreated. On one hand, CLLs can produce mediastinal shift,

Disclosures: The authors have nothing to disclose.
[a] Department of Surgery, University of CA - San Francisco, 513 Parnassus Avenue, S-321, San Francisco, CA 94143, USA; [b] Division of Pediatric Surgery, Department of Surgery, University of CA - San Francisco, 550 16th Street, 5th Floor, UCSF Box 0570, San Francisco, CA 94143, USA
* Corresponding author.
E-mail address: jarrett.moyer@ucsf.edu

Clin Perinatol 44 (2017) 781–794
http://dx.doi.org/10.1016/j.clp.2017.08.003
perinatology.theclinics.com

polyhydramnios, and fetal nonimmune hydrops in 5% to 30% of cases,[2,3] requiring prenatal intervention to avoid fetal demise. On the other hand, approximately 1 in 5 cases are diagnosed outside of the neonatal period incidentally or because of infection or pneumothorax.[4] Finally, in utero behavior of CLLs is variable, with an early proliferative phase producing a peak in size around 25 weeks' gestation, often followed by size regression in the third trimester. In a case series of 600 CLLs, 68% of pulmonary sequestration and 15% of CPAM underwent marked spontaneous regression before birth.[2] Accordingly, the rarity of CLLs, heterogeneity in lesion histology for prenatally diagnosed lung lesions, and an unpredictable and widely variable natural history make the development of evidence-based treatment algorithms difficult. Thus, although the development of hydrops mandates prenatal intervention, and symptomatic neonates clearly benefit from resection, optimal treatment of the asymptomatic CLL is less clear and is determined on a case-by-case basis with the guidance of case series and expert opinion.

In patients who warrant surgical intervention, formal lobectomy is recommended over segmental resection.[5,6] Case reports and series have demonstrated precursors to mucinous bronchioloalveolar carcinoma harbored in CPAM type 1[7,8]; PPB can be indistinguishable from CPAM type 4, resulting in inadequate surgical margins and risk of recurrence with segmental resection.[9] Additionally, determining lesion margins both preoperatively on CT scan and intraoperatively is difficult, resulting in a high risk of incomplete resection with nonanatomic resection.[4,5] Traditionally, lobectomy occurred as an open surgical procedure through posterolateral thoracotomy. However, Albanese and colleagues[10] first described a completely thoracoscopic minimally invasive lobectomy in 2003. Subsequent case series and a meta-analysis have shown the thoracoscopic technique to provide improved or equivalent complication rates, decreased hospital length of stay, and decreased time of tube thoracostomy when compared with open techniques.[11–15] The focus of this article is on the indications, surgical approach, technical considerations, postoperative care, and outcomes of thoracoscopic resection of CLLs, in particular CPAM.

INDICATIONS/CONTRAINDICATIONS

As mentioned earlier, the clinical presentation of antenatally diagnosed CLLs varies widely, from fetal nonimmune hydrops to asymptomatic term live birth extending into childhood. Large lesions can produce mediastinal shift, cardiac compression, and obstruction of the vena cava, resulting in profound hemodynamic alterations and development of hydrops in the fetus. Lesions can be risk stratified according to the cystic adenomatoid volume ratio (CVR), which normalizes lesion volume to head circumference and predicts an 80% risk of hydrops for a CVR greater than 1.6.[16,17] Fetuses with a CVR greater than 1.6 should be monitored with weekly ultrasound examinations, as hydrops is associated with near 100% fetal mortality if left untreated.[3,18] Treatment strategies include maternal betamethasone administration as well as invasive techniques, such as fetal lobectomy via maternal laparotomy and hysterotomy, thoracoamniotic shunting, radiofrequency or laser ablation, or percutaneous ultrasound-guided sclerotherapy.[19] Steroid administration is especially effective in treating microcystic lesions producing nonimmune hydrops, with survival rates to delivery as high as 92%.[20–22] Given the effectiveness of prenatal steroids in the treatment of hydrops, there are now fewer clinical scenarios whereby invasive fetal intervention is indicated.

Most fetuses with a prenatal diagnosis of CLL proceed to live birth without the development of hydrops. Of these neonates, roughly one-quarter will be symptomatic at birth with abnormal breathing and respiratory distress, with large lesions portending a higher risk.[2,23] Symptomatic neonates should proceed to surgical resection, which may be facilitated by ex utero intrapartum therapy (EXIT) or support with extracorporeal membrane oxygenation (ECMO) in rare cases of severe distress.[1,2]

The timing and necessity of surgical resection of CLLs in asymptomatic neonates is a source of controversy. Roughly 10% to 30% of asymptomatic neonates will develop an infection within the first year of life,[4,24] and the presence of infectious symptoms correlates with higher rates of intraoperative and postoperative complications and longer hospitalizations.[4,25] Additionally, early surgical resection offers the theoretic advantage of compensatory lung growth.[26,27] However, in a long-term prospective study, there was no correlation between age at operation and eventual pulmonary function or exercise capacity following lobectomy.[28] Finally, some investigators advocate early resection because of the risk of malignancy, namely, difficulty in distinguishing CPAM from PPB and the observation that CPAM type 1 can harbor precursors to mucinous bronchioloalveolar carcinoma that can undergo malignant transformation later in life.[8] The authors' institution has developed a protocol for asymptomatic neonates with CLLs, which includes chest CT scan at 6 months of age to allow for better evaluation of the location of the lesion and lobectomy at 6 to 9 months of age for those with a higher risk of future respiratory infections (radiographic findings of predominantly large cysts).

After determining the need for and timing of surgical resection for CLLs, it is important to consider whether a thoracoscopic approach is feasible for resection. Although case series and a meta-analysis have shown no difference in thoracoscopic complication rates compared with open resection,[11–14] case series demonstrate conversion rates as high as 33% to 50%[11,29] with early experience. The primary risk factor for conversion to open thoracotomy is the presence of preoperative respiratory symptoms and infection,[11,29,30] which can produce intrathoracic adhesions and a potentially more difficult dissection. Resection should be performed after resolution of the acute infection and inflammation. Once infection subsides, an initial thoracoscopic approach seems to be safe, as a recent case series of lung resections in the setting of CLLs and preoperative infection found no difference in complication rates between open and thoracoscopic approaches.[31] Additional risk factors for intraoperative conversion to thoracotomy may include procedures performed early in the surgeon's learning curve,[29] with one case series demonstrating an early conversion rate of 27% reduced to 8% with increased surgeon experience,[30] and patient age, as another series found a higher rate of conversion in patients less than 5 months of age at lobectomy.[14] However, multiple series have shown no difference in complication or conversion rates based on patient age or size.[32–34]

SURGICAL CONSIDERATIONS
Preoperative Planning

Most CLLs are diagnosed prenatally, with surgical timing and planning dependent on the presence or absence of respiratory distress or altered breathing at birth. Lesions with CVR greater than 0.84 are at an increased risk for respiratory symptoms at birth,[23] and some investigators advocate delivery at a quaternary care center for lesions with a CVR greater than 1.0.[35] This practice facilitates resection during the EXIT procedure or ECMO support as a bridge to resection. In the absence of severe respiratory distress, a thorough postnatal preoperative workup should be performed, which includes advanced cross-sectional imaging with contrast-enhanced chest CT scan.[1] CT allows increased definition of the lung lesion and its location relative to surrounding anatomic structures, which may help narrow the differential diagnosis.

Patient Positioning

Proper patient positioning for thoracoscopic lung resections allows optimal ergonomics for the operating surgeon, excellent visualization of the hemithorax and pulmonary hilum, and protects patients from pressure- or stretch-induced injury. To achieve this, patients are first placed on the operating table supine, to allow for safe induction of general anesthesia with optimal oropharyngeal access for the anesthesiologist. After induction of anesthesia, intubation should proceed to allow for single lung ventilation. This ventilation can be achieved through main stem intubation with or without the use of a fiber optic bronchoscope; other techniques include insertion of a bronchial block or simultaneous main stem intubation with 2 endotracheal tubes.[36] The method for single lung ventilation depends on the expertise of the pediatric anesthesiologist and the size and age of the patients. Double lumen endotracheal tubes are used for older patients. Once the airway is secure, the authors place patients in the lateral decubitus position. Care is taken to position the head, neck, arms, hips, and legs in neutral positions with all pressure points protected by padding. The surgeon and the assistant stand on the same side of the table, facing the patients' anterior chest and abdomen, with the thoracoscopic monitor placed opposite the operating surgeon, as demonstrated in **Fig. 1**.

Surgical Approach

The authors prefer a completely thoracoscopic approach and formal lobectomy for treatment of CLLs. Three trocars are inserted to accommodate the camera and 2 working instruments. A 12-mm port allows passage of a laparoscopic stapler as well as removal of the complete resected lobe for thorough histopathologic analysis. Variations to this approach include a hybrid procedure that uses a mini thoracotomy for direct manipulation and removal of the specimen as well as pulverization of the resected specimen to facilitate removal.[37] The authors find the 12-mm port enables specimen retrieval, while maintaining the benefits of minimally invasive approaches, including improved cosmesis and shorter hospital length of stay.[11]

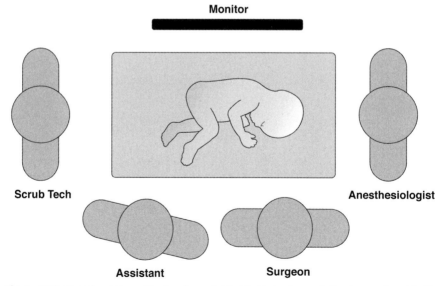

Fig. 1. Patient and room positioning for a right-sided lobectomy. Patients are placed in the lateral decubitus position, facing the surgeon and assistant. The thorax is aligned between the surgeon and the monitor.

Most investigators recommend formal lobectomy rather than wedge resection for the treatment of CLLs.[1] Retrospective case series have demonstrated contrast-enhanced CT has low sensitivity for identification of multiple lesions within the same lobe,[5] leaving local approaches prone to incomplete resection and residual disease. Accordingly, a meta-analysis showed a 15% risk of incomplete resection with nonanatomic resections,[4] compared with 0% with lobectomy. Additionally, case reports of early occurrence of PPB after local CLL resection[9] likely reflect incomplete resection rather than malignant transformation, illustrating the difficulty in obtaining a definitive preoperative diagnosis and the danger of obtaining inadequate surgical margins. Finally, children who undergo formal lobectomy have good pulmonary functional outcomes, with most patients achieving normal exercise capacity and pulmonary function.[28] However, formal lobectomy is not always feasible; lesions in multiple lobes may necessitate local resection.

Surgical Procedure

The following description of the surgical procedure focuses on younger patients less than 1 year of age at the authors' institution. After induction of anesthesia, sterile preparation and draping of the entire hemithorax of interest, and administration of prophylactic antibiotics, the surgical procedure begins. Access to the thoracic cavity is achieved by placement of 3 to 4 thoracoscopic trocars, as shown in **Fig. 2**. After instillation of subcutaneous bupivacaine, the authors first place a Veress needle with a radially expanding sheath anteroinferior to the inferior angle of the scapula and insufflate the chest with 4 torr carbon

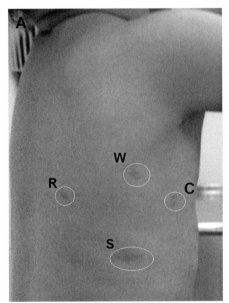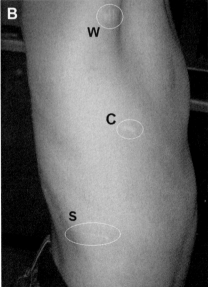

Fig. 2. (*A*) Incisions illustrating port placement for a lower lobectomy. The camera is initially inserted through the incision anteroinferior to the tip of the scapula (W) and is then moved to the mid axillary (C) line to allow triangulation of the lower lobe. The inferior port is enlarged to 12 mm to facilitate the stapler and specimen retrieval (S). A fourth incision (R) can be made to assist in lung retraction for large cystic lesions. (*B*) Port placement for a right upper lobectomy. The initial incision (C) remains the camera port, while a working port (W) is placed cranially to allow triangulation of the lesion. The inferior working port is again enlarged to 12 mm (S).

dioxide insufflation at 1.0 L/min to create a pneumothorax and collapse the lung completely. The Veress needle is removed, and a 5-mm port is placed through the sheath to facilitate a 4-mm, 30° telescope. Two 5-mm working ports are then placed along the midanterior axillary line. A fourth port may be placed to allow improved retraction and hilar exposure for lesions with large cystic components, as shown in **Fig. 2**A. These ports allow the use of a 3-mm, 20-cm monopolar hook cautery, atraumatic grasper, Maryland dissector, and curved scissors as well as a 5-mm or 3-mm laparoscopic vessel-sealing device. Placement of the 5-mm port in the anterior axillary line occurs at the level of the fissure, to allow dissection along this plane; enlargement of this port to 12 mm facilitates use of the laparoscopic stapler, if used, to divide the bronchus and the fissure if incomplete. Rothenberg and colleagues[37] also describes the recent use of a 5-mm stapler that may facilitate stapling in small neonates. Other techniques include a hybrid procedure, including a mini-posterolateral thoracotomy in the fifth intercostal space, using a muscle-sparing approach and two to three 3- to 5-mm trocars.[38]

The lobar dissection begins with mobilization of the lung, releasing the inferior pulmonary ligament and any pleuropulmonary adhesions. In cases of intralobar bronchopulmonary sequestration, the systemic vascular supply is identified, ligated, and divided. Once the lung is free, attention is turned to the hilum. The branches of the superior or inferior pulmonary vein are dissected free but not divided in order to avoid vascular congestion, as shown in **Fig. 3**. The authors then complete the fissure with the vessel-sealing device before dissecting the pulmonary arterial supply, as demonstrated in **Fig. 4**. Once the vascular supply is isolated, the arterial branches, seen in **Fig. 5**, and then the veins are sealed and divided with the vessel-sealing device. Middle lobectomies proceed first with completion of the fissures to allow identification of the branches of both the pulmonary vein and artery, followed by isolation and division of segmental branches using the vessel-sealing device. Other strategies for sealing and dividing vessels include endoscopic clips and use of the stapler, though these approaches are sometimes limited by patient size in small infants and neonates.

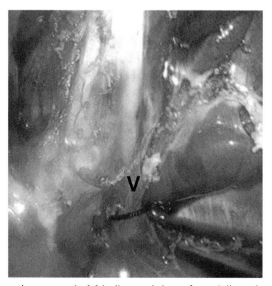

Fig. 3. The inferior pulmonary vein (V) is dissected circumferentially and encircled with a silk tie. The tie can aid in the arterial dissection and can provide traction on the vein during division using the vessel sealing device.

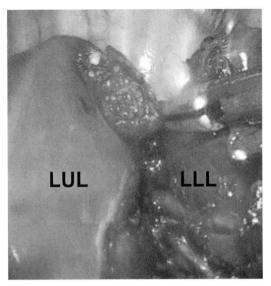

Fig. 4. The 5 mm vessel-sealing device is used to complete the oblique fissure of the left lung, isolating the left lower lobe (LLL) from the left upper lobe (LUL).

Placement of traction silk sutures around vessels before division may facilitate exposure and aid in safe division, especially in infants less than 15 kg.[39] Finally, to divide the bronchus, the authors enlarge one of the 5-mm working ports to 12 mm to facilitate laparoscopic stapler. If necessary, the fissure can also be completed with the stapler. In cases whereby the hemithorax is too small to facilitate a 12-mm port and stapler, the authors divide the bronchus sharply and oversew the bronchial stump using

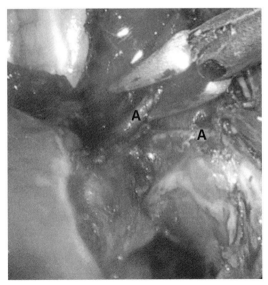

Fig. 5. The left lower lobe segmental arterial branches (A) are isolated and divided using the LigaSure.

interrupted sutures. The specimen is removed intact through the 12-mm incision, which may need to be enlarged slightly to allow specimen removal. A thoracostomy tube is inserted through the most inferior port site, and the lung is reexpanded under direct visualization. Port site incisions are then closed in 2 layers, using an absorbable suture.

COMPLICATIONS AND MANAGEMENT

Thoracoscopic resection of CLL can incur both intraoperative and postoperative complications. However, multiple case series have demonstrated a low incidence of overall morbidity, as described in **Table 1**, and no difference in complication rates between minimally invasive and open approaches to resection.[11,13–15] In their meta-analysis, Nasr and colleagues[12] found a 21% rate of overall morbidity and a 16% rate of respiratory complications, most commonly postoperative pneumonia. The most frequently described intraoperative complications include hemorrhage requiring transfusion, bronchial injury requiring repair, phrenic nerve injury, and incomplete resection of the lesion. Common postoperative complications include pneumonia, persistent air leak/pneumothorax, and need for blood transfusion.

Additionally, although not a true complication, the most common unanticipated intraoperative event is conversion to an open procedure. Various centers report different rates of conversion, ranging from 1% to 50%.[11,29,37,40] As mentioned earlier, one established risk factor for conversion is the presence of preoperative infectious symptoms, and conversion rates are lower in asymptomatic patients.[11,29] Other factors that may increase the risk for conversion are procedures done early in the surgeon learning curve[29,30] and patient age less than 5 months,[14] though multiple series have demonstrated high rates of thoracoscopic success in small neonates.[32,33] In general, the surgeon should consider conversion to an open procedure when unable to safely visualize, dissect, delineate, and divide hilar structures. Specific barriers to safe hilar dissection include pleural adhesions, aberrant hilar anatomy, incomplete fissure, and hemorrhage.

Specific Complications

Intraoperative
Hemorrhage Sources of bleeding during thoracoscopic dissection include intercostal vascular injury, inflammatory pleural adhesions, and injury to hilar vessels. Although not immediately life threatening, bleeding from inflammatory adhesions can result in acute blood loss anemia requiring blood transfusion and can prevent visualization of hilar structures, resulting in conversion to an open procedure. The meticulous use of electrocautery and the LigaSure can reduce oozing from these adhesions. Following basic surgical principles, hilar vessels should be identified and controlled circumferentially before attempts at division. Incidental injury to these vessels incurred during dissection or division can produce life-threatening hemorrhage. Methods for controlling a vascular injury include local pressure, suture repair, and ligation; these injuries often require emergent conversion to thoracotomy.

Bronchial injury Although rare, thermal injury, staple injury, or laceration to an adjacent or incorrectly identified bronchus or bronchiole can lead to major morbidity, including complementary lobectomy.[34] If identified intraoperatively, successful primary suture repair has been described after conversion to an open procedure.[38] Missed injuries result in a prolonged air leak and often necessitate reoperation for bronchial or bronchiolar repair.

Table 1
Perioperative complications

Author	n	Morbidity (%)	Infection (%)	Bleeding/ Transfusion (%)	Prolonged Tube Thoracostomy (%)	Pneumothorax (%)	Prolonged Intubation (%)	Phrenic Nerve Injury (%)	Chylothorax (%)	Bronchial Injury (%)
Albanese & Rothenberg,[40] 2007	144	4 (2.8)	2 (1.4)	0	1 (0.7)	1 (0.7)	0	0	0	0
Seong et al,[30] 2013	50	8 (16)	0	1 (2.0)	6 (12)	0	0	0	1 (2.0)	0
Kunisaki et al,[14] 2014	49	15 (31)	0	11 (22)	2 (4.1)	0	0	2 (4.1)	1 (2.0)	0
Boubnova et al,[34] 2011	30	11 (37)	4 (13)	2 (6.7)	4 (13)	0	0	0	0	1 (3.3)
Kaneko et al,[33] 2010	16	4 (25)	0	0	1 (6.3)	0	2 (13)	1 (6.3)	0	0
Rahman & Lakhoo,[13] 2009	14	2 (14)	0	2 (14)	0	0	0	0	0	0
Diamond et al,[15] 2007	12	4 (33)	3 (25)	0	0	1 (8.3)	0	0	0	0

Incomplete resection The risk of incomplete resection depends on the surgical approach, with nonanatomic resections demonstrating a 15% risk, compared with 0% with formal lobectomy.[4] This risk may be due to the observed low sensitivity of contrast-enhanced CT scan for identifying secondary lesions in the affected lobe.[5] In cases of residual disease identified on postoperative pathology, reoperation should be considered to gain clear margins or to perform formal lobectomy. If residual disease is missed, cases thought to be CLLs can manifest PPB[9] and CPAM type 1 can undergo eventual malignant transformation into bronchioloalveolar carcinoma.[7,8]

Postoperative
Persistent air leak/pneumothorax Most case series report rates of persistent air leaks and pneumothorax less than 10%.[12,33,34] Air leaks can originate at the bronchial staple/suture line, a transected bronchiole, or a missed injury to an adjacent bronchus. Small air leaks will often resolve with continued thoracostomy drainage. However, if the lung fails to fully expand or the air leak does not resolve, reoperation may be necessary to identify and address bronchial or bronchiolar injury.

Pneumonia Approximately 5% to 10% of patients develop postoperative pneumonia following thoracoscopic lung resection.[12] Initial treatment is with intravenous antibiotics while obtaining imaging to assess for undrained pleural effusions that may become infected. Any undrained collections should be drained, and development of purulent drainage may require reoperation and chest washout.

POSTOPERATIVE CARE

Generally, neonates and infants do well after thoracoscopic resection of CLL. Following completion of the case, patients without preoperative respiratory distress are usually extubated in the operating room. The thoracostomy tube is maintained in place until there is no air leak and no pneumothorax on chest radiograph, usually 1 to 3 days.[11,12,15,38] Patients may restart normal oral intake after recovery from general anesthesia.[10] Postoperative pain control is most often achieved with a combination of oral and intravenous analgesics, with the rare need for regional analgesia through placement of an epidural. In the uncomplicated case, neonates and infants are ready to return home within 2 to 8 days.[11,30,34] In a large case series including 97 thoracoscopic lung resections, Rothenberg reported an average postoperative hospital length of stay of 2.4 days.[38]

OUTCOMES

In addition to the low rates of major perioperative morbidity described earlier and in **Table 1**, long-term functional outcomes are excellent following lobectomy in children. In a combined prospective and retrospective analysis of 15 children undergoing lobectomy for CLLs before 1 year of age, Beres and colleagues[26] showed normal forced vital capacity in 93%, normal forced expiratory volume in 1 second in 86%, and normal diffusion capacity in 100% of children at 5 years of age or older. Additionally, Naito and colleagues[28] demonstrated excellent long-term pulmonary function and exercise capacity in children undergoing lobectomy, with no correlation between age at lobectomy and exercise capacity or pulmonary function results. However, both of these series included children who underwent open thoracotomy; no study has examined long-term pulmonary function in patients undergoing thoracoscopic lobectomy exclusively.

SUMMARY

CLLs comprise a heterogeneous group of developmental and histologic entities and are often diagnosed on screening prenatal ultrasound. Although large lesions can produce hemodynamic compromise and fetal nonimmune hydrops or neonatal respiratory distress, most fetuses with CLLs proceed to uncomplicated term vaginal delivery and are asymptomatic at birth. The potential risk for developing malignancy and infectious complications drives the decision to resect CLLs in asymptomatic patients. Accordingly, prophylactic surgery should entail minimal morbidity and excellent long-term outcomes. Since first described in 2003,[10] thoracoscopic lobectomy for CLLs has been shown to provide decreased hospital length of stay and decreased time of tube thoracostomy when compared with open resection, without increased risk of perioperative morbidity.[11–15] Additionally, most children exhibit normal long-term pulmonary function following resection.[26,28] The surgical technique continues to evolve, with outcomes improving as surgeons gain more experience.[30,37] Recent advances in minimally invasive instrumentation, including the development of a 5-mm endoscopic stapler, promise to address some of the remaining challenges of thoracoscopic surgery in small infants and neonates.[37]

Best Practices

What is the current practice?

Thoracoscopic lobectomy for congenital lung lesions

Best practice/guideline/care path objectives:

- Follow prenatally diagnosed CLLs with serial sonographic assessment and calculation of CVR.
- Administer maternal betamethasone for large CLL (CVR >1.6) and to reverse hydrops.
- Resect symptomatic CLLs in the neonatal period.
- Obtain contrast-enhanced chest CT before resection in asymptomatic patients.
- Resect asymptomatic CLLs before the onset of respiratory symptoms.
- Formal lobectomy is superior to wedge resection for unilobar CLLs.
- Thoracoscopic resection is a safe and feasible approach in children with CLLs.
- Send surgical specimens for pathologic analysis to rule out occult malignancy and confirm the diagnosis.

What changes in current practice are likely to improve outcomes?

- Development and application of infection risk-stratification methods to assist in determining the optimal timing of prophylactic thoracoscopy
- Further improvements in endoscopic instrumentation to facilitate resection in small neonates
- Improved understanding of the impact of surgical timing on long-term pulmonary function

Major recommendations

- The CVR is a reproducible prenatal prognostic tool for predicting the development of hydrops and/or respiratory symptoms at birth.
- Prenatal maternal betamethasone administration is indicated to decrease the size of large microcystic CLLs and reverse hydrops.
- Symptomatic CLLs should be resected in the neonatal period.
- Contrast-enhanced chest CT is the best imaging study for postnatal assessment of CLLs.
- Asymptomatic CLLs should be treated on a case-by-case basis, with delayed resection (6–9 months) reasonable in patients with low infection risk and no features concerning for malignancy.
- Formal lobectomy is superior to segmentectomy in the treatment of unilobar CLLs.
- Thoracoscopic resection is a safe and feasible option in selected children with CLLs, particularly those without previous infection.

Summary statement

Symptomatic CLLs require prompt management in both the prenatal and neonatal periods. However, most CLLs do not produce symptoms, and infection and malignancy risk is low; thus, timing of resection is controversial. In most cases of unilobar CLLs that proceed to resection, thoracoscopic formal lobectomy is the optimal treatment approach.

Data from Refs.[1–5,18]

REFERENCES

1. Baird R, Puligandla PS, Laberge J-M. Congenital lung malformations: informing best practice. Semin Pediatr Surg 2014;23(5):270–7.
2. Adzick NS. Management of fetal lung lesions. Clin Perinatol 2009;36(2):363–76.
3. Cavoretto P, Molina F, Poggi S, et al. Prenatal diagnosis and outcome of echogenic fetal lung lesions. Ultrasound Obstet Gynecol 2008;32(6):769–83.
4. Stanton M, Njere I, Ade-Ajayi N, et al. Systematic review and meta-analysis of the postnatal management of congenital cystic lung lesions. J Pediatr Surg 2009; 44(5):1027–33.
5. Muller CO, Berrebi D, Kheniche A, et al. Is radical lobectomy required in congenital cystic adenomatoid malformation? J Pediatr Surg 2012;47(4):642–5.
6. Khosa JK, Leong SL, Borzi PA. Congenital cystic adenomatoid malformation of the lung: indications and timing of surgery. Pediatr Surg Int 2004;20(7):505–8.
7. Lantuejoul S, Nicholson AG, Sartori G, et al. Mucinous cells in type 1 pulmonary congenital cystic adenomatoid malformation as mucinous bronchioloalveolar carcinoma precursors. Am J Surg Pathol 2007;31(6):961–9.
8. Ramos SG, Barbosa GH, Tavora FR, et al. Bronchioloalveolar carcinoma arising in a congenital pulmonary airway malformation in a child: case report with an update of this association. J Pediatr Surg 2007;42(5):e1–4.
9. Papagiannopoulos KA, Sheppard M, Bush AP, et al. Pleuropulmonary blastoma: is prophylactic resection of congenital lung cysts effective? Ann Thorac Surg 2001;72(2):604–5.
10. Albanese CT, Sydorak RM, Tsao K, et al. Thoracoscopic lobectomy for prenatally diagnosed lung lesions. J Pediatr Surg 2003;38(4):553–5.
11. Vu LT, Farmer DL, Nobuhara KK, et al. Thoracoscopic versus open resection for congenital cystic adenomatoid malformations of the lung. J Pediatr Surg 2008; 43(1):35–9.
12. Nasr A, Bass J. Thoracoscopic vs open resection of congenital lung lesions: a meta-analysis. J Pediatr Surg 2012;47(5):857–61.
13. Rahman N, Lakhoo K. Comparison between open and thoracoscopic resection of congenital lung lesions. J Pediatr Surg 2009;44(2):333–6.
14. Kunisaki SM, Powelson IA, Haydar B, et al. Thoracoscopic vs open lobectomy in infants and young children with congenital lung malformations. J Am Coll Surg 2014;218(2):261–70.
15. Diamond IR, Herrera P, Langer JC, et al. Thoracoscopic versus open resection of congenital lung lesions: a case-matched study. J Pediatr Surg 2007;42(6): 1057–61.
16. Crombleholme TM, Coleman B, Hedrick H, et al. Cystic adenomatoid malformation volume ratio predicts outcome in prenatally diagnosed cystic adenomatoid malformation of the lung. J Pediatr Surg 2002;37(3):331–8.

17. Yong PJ, Von Dadelszen P, Carpara D, et al. Prediction of pediatric outcome after prenatal diagnosis and expectant antenatal management of congenital cystic adenomatoid malformation. Fetal Diagn Ther 2012;31(2):94–102.
18. Adzick NS, Harrison MR, Crombleholme TM, et al. Fetal lung lesions: management and outcome. Am J Obstet Gynecol 1998;179(4):884–9. Available at: http://www.ncbi.nlm.nih.gov/pubmed/9790364. Accessed March 1, 2017.
19. Puligandla PS, Laberge J-M. Congenital lung lesions. Clin Perinatol 2012;39(2): 331–47.
20. Tsao K, Hawgood S, Vu L, et al. Resolution of hydrops fetalis in congenital cystic adenomatoid malformation after prenatal steroid therapy. J Pediatr Surg 2003; 38(3):508–10.
21. Curran PF, Jelin EB, Rand L, et al. Prenatal steroids for microcystic congenital cystic adenomatoid malformations. J Pediatr Surg 2010;45(1):145–50.
22. Loh KC, Jelin E, Hirose S, et al. Microcystic congenital pulmonary airway malformation with hydrops fetalis: steroids vs open fetal resection. J Pediatr Surg 2012; 47(1):36–9.
23. Ruchonnet–Metrailler I, Leroy–Terquem E, Stirnemann J, et al. Neonatal outcomes of prenatally diagnosed congenital pulmonary malformations. Pediatrics 2014; 133(5). Available at: http://pediatrics.aappublications.org/content/133/5/e1285. short. Accessed September 7, 2017.
24. Aziz D, Langer JC, Tuuha SE, et al. Perinatally diagnosed asymptomatic congenital cystic adenomatoid malformation: to resect or not? J Pediatr Surg 2004;39(3): 329–34 [discussion: 329–34]. Available at: http://www.ncbi.nlm.nih.gov/pubmed/ 15017547. Accessed March 14, 2017.
25. Aspirot A, Puligandla PS, Bouchard S, et al. A contemporary evaluation of surgical outcome in neonates and infants undergoing lung resection. J Pediatr Surg 2008;43(3):508–12.
26. Beres A, Aspirot A, Paris C, et al. A contemporary evaluation of pulmonary function in children undergoing lung resection in infancy. J Pediatr Surg 2011;46(5): 829–32.
27. Komori K, Kamagata S, Hirobe S, et al. Radionuclide imaging study of long-term pulmonary function after lobectomy in children with congenital cystic lung disease. J Pediatr Surg 2009;44(11):2096–100.
28. Naito Y, Beres A, Lapidus-Krol E, et al. Does earlier lobectomy result in better long-term pulmonary function in children with congenital lung anomalies? A prospective study. J Pediatr Surg 2012;47(5):852–6.
29. Garrett-Cox R, MacKinlay G, Munro F, et al. Early experience of pediatric thoracoscopic lobectomy in the UK. J Laparoendosc Adv Surg Tech A 2008;18(3): 457–9.
30. Seong YW, Kang CH, Kim J-T, et al. Video-assisted thoracoscopic lobectomy in children: safety, efficacy, and risk factors for conversion to thoracotomy. Ann Thorac Surg 2013;95(4):1236–42.
31. Sueyoshi R, Koga H, Suzuki K, et al. Surgical intervention for congenital pulmonary airway malformation (CPAM) patients with preoperative pneumonia and abscess formation: "open versus thoracoscopic lobectomy". Pediatr Surg Int 2016; 32(4):347–51.
32. Rothenberg SS, Kuenzler KA, Middlesworth W, et al. Thoracoscopic lobectomy in infants less than 10 Kg with prenatally diagnosed cystic lung disease. J Laparoendosc Adv Surg Tech A 2011;21(2):181–4.
33. Kaneko K, Ono Y, Tainaka T, et al. Thoracoscopic lobectomy for congenital cystic lung diseases in neonates and small infants. Pediatr Surg Int 2010;26(4):361–5.

34. Boubnova J, Peycelon M, Garbi O, et al. Thoracoscopy in the management of congenital lung diseases in infancy. Surg Endosc 2011;25(2):593–6.

35. Ehrenberg-Buchner S, Stapf AM, Berman DR, et al. Fetal lung lesions: can we start to breathe easier? Am J Obstet Gynecol 2013;208(2):151.e1-7.

36. Hammer GB, Fitzmaurice BG, Brodsky JB. Methods for single-lung ventilation in pediatric patients. Anesth Analg 1999;89(6):1426.

37. Rothenberg SS, Middlesworth W, Kadennhe-Chiweshe A, et al. Two decades of experience with thoracoscopic lobectomy in infants and children: standardizing techniques for advanced thoracoscopic surgery. J Laparoendosc Adv Surg Tech A 2015;25(5):423–8.

38. Rothenberg SS. First decade's experience with thoracoscopic lobectomy in infants and children. J Pediatr Surg 2008;43(1):40–5.

39. Koga H, Suzuki K, Nishimura K, et al. Traction sutures allow endoscopic staples to be used safely during thoracoscopic pulmonary lobectomy in children weighing less than 15 kg. J Laparoendosc Adv Surg Tech A 2013;23(1):81–3.

40. Albanese CT, Rothenberg SS. Experience with 144 consecutive pediatric thoracoscopic lobectomies. J Laparoendosc Adv Surg Tech A 2007;17(3):339–41.

Fundoplication

Bethany J. Slater, MD*, Steven S. Rothenberg, MD

KEYWORDS

- Children - Fundoplication - Gastroesophageal reflux - Minimally invasive - Nissen
- Pediatrics - Reflux

KEY POINTS

- There are several diagnostic tools for infants with GERD, such as upper gastrointestinal series, pH probe testing, and impedance studies.
- The key technical aspects of laparoscopic Nissen fundoplication include creation of an adequate intra-abdominal esophagus, minimal dissection of the hiatus with exposure of the right crus to identify the gastroesophageal junction, crural repair, and creation of floppy, 360° wrap that is oriented at the 11-o'clock position.
- There are several controversial aspects regarding the management of GERD, including the indications and timing of surgical management, optimal patient selection, and technical modifications to prevent recurrence.

INTRODUCTION

Gastroesophageal reflux is defined as the passage of gastric contents into the esophagus. Gastroesophageal reflux disease (GERD) refers to the pathologic symptoms and complications that result from reflux. GERD is a common condition and affects approximately 7% to 20% of the pediatric population.[1] Several physiologic barriers exist to prevent reflux from the stomach into the lower esophagus, such as the lower esophageal sphincter, the angle of His, and the length of the intra-abdominal esophagus. In addition, mechanisms are present to both minimize the amount of reflux in the esophagus, such as esophageal peristalsis, and to limit esophageal injury, such as saliva and other enzymes.[2] The adverse effects of GERD occur from the failure of 1 or more of these factors. Transient lower esophageal sphincter relaxation is the most important pathophysiologic mechanism leading to GERD.[3] In neonates, the lower esophageal sphincter is often immature, leading to reflux. In addition, several

Disclosure Statement: Dr B.J. Slater has no commercial or financial conflicts of interest. Dr S.S. Rothenberg is a consultant for JustRight Surgical. His role is not in conflict with this article. No products from JustRight Surgical are used for the technique described. No funding sources have been used for this article.
Pediatric Surgery, Rocky Mountain Hospital for Children, 2055 High Street, Suite 370, Denver, CO 80205, USA
* Corresponding author.
E-mail address: Bjslater1@gmail.com

congenital anomalies also increase the risk of GERD in infants, including esophageal atresia and congenital diaphragmatic hernia.

CLINICAL PRESENTATION

In infants, typical symptoms of GERD in include regurgitation, emesis, poor weight gain, and food refusal.[4,5] Pulmonary symptoms, such as coughing, wheezing, choking, apnea, and apparent life-threatening events (ALTEs), can also be the presenting symptoms of GERD. Distinguishing normal regurgitation from more problematic symptoms can be difficult in infants.

DIAGNOSIS

Several diagnostic tests may be used to detect both the presence and absence of reflux as well as rule out other pathologies. Upper gastrointestinal radiography can identify reflux in approximately half of the patients and delineates the anatomy of esophagus and upper gastrointestinal tract. The level of reflux and presence of a hiatal hernia can be evaluated on upper gastrointestinal radiography. The most useful aspect of this test, however, is to rule out other anatomic abnormalities of the upper gastrointestinal tract, such as malrotation. A 24-hour PH probe testing has been considered the gold standard for diagnosing GERD since the 1980s. This study is performed by placing electrodes in the distal esophagus and measuring the pH. A score is calculated from the time the pH is less than 4, total number of reflux episodes, number of episodes greater than 5 minutes, and the longest reflux episode. There are some limitations to this study, and patients must be off of acid suppression medications before testing. Impedance studies, in which multichannel electrode pairs are placed in the esophagus and stomach detecting the flow of gastric contents, are used more frequently because they measure nonacidic reflux and can be performed while children are on antireflux medications.[6] Adding impedance monitoring can thus improve sensitivity for the detection of GERD.

Other diagnostic evaluations, such as upper endoscopy with biopsies, bronchoscopy with bronchial washings, and gastric emptying studies, may also be used to add further confirmatory information or when a diagnosis is unclear. These studies are usually unnecessary, however, when evaluating infants.

CLINICAL MANAGEMENT

The treatment of pathologic GERD typically starts with dietary modifications and postural changes. For infants, elevation of the head of the bed and frequent, small-volume meals with thickened formulas or agents are generally recommended. Next, pharmacologic agents may be added consisting of antireflux medication and prokinetic agents. The main acid-suppressant agents used for GERD are H_2-receptor antagonists and proton pump inhibitors. Motility medications, such as metoclopramide, have been widely used although studies demonstrating their efficacy have been limited.[7]

INDICATIONS

Indications for operative management include failure of medical therapy with poor weight gain or failure to thrive (FTT), continued respiratory symptoms, and esophagitis. Situations in which a trial of medical treatment may not be necessary include infants who present with ALTEs and no other identifiable etiology. In addition, neurologically impaired infants who require a gastrostomy for feeding and concerns for aspiration may also benefit from a fundoplication at the same time.

Although reflux often improves in infants in 6 months to a year, adverse events can occur from pathologic GERD in the meantime. In addition to ALTEs or FTT, infants can develop chronic lung disease and oral aversion. There are very low morbidity and good outcomes for laparoscopic fundoplication in infants. Early intervention for GERD may potentially avoid or minimize the use of feeding tubes, complications from reflux, and long-term respiratory and feeding issues.

TECHNIQUE

The laparoscopic Nissen fundoplication is the most common procedure performed. This technique has been developed over the past 2 decades with minor revisions to improve outcome.[8–10]

- Preparation and patient positioning: the patient is placed at the end of the table with the surgeon at the foot of the table (**Fig. 1**). The legs are placed in a frog-leg position.
- The monitor is placed over the patient's head and an orogastric tube is placed by the anesthesiologist.
- Trocar position: five trocars are inserted with the camera port at the umbilicus, working ports in the right quadrant and left midquadrant, a liver retractor port in the right midquadrant in the midclavicular line to the patient's right of the falciform, and a stomach retractor in the left upper quadrant.
- The left upper quadrant trocar position should be the gastrostomy tube site if one is to be performed and may be marked before insufflation to assure that the button is far enough from the costal margin (**Fig. 2**). Otherwise, the port should be placed at the costal margin in the midclavicular line.

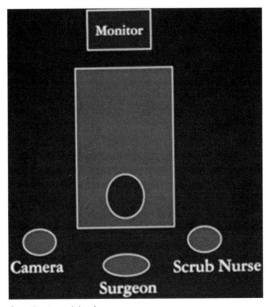

Fig. 1. Schematic of patient positioning.

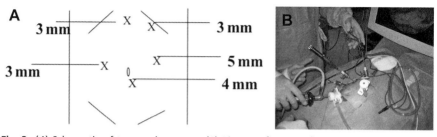

Fig. 2. (*A*) Schematic of trocar placement. (*B*) Picture of trocar placement.

- Insufflation pressures may be between 12 mm Hg to 15 mm Hg depending on the size and medical condition of the patient.
- Surgical approach: the left lobe of the liver is retracted superiorly to expose the gastroesophageal junction through the right upper quadrant port.
  - Although a self-retaining retractor may be used, a Babcock retractor with a locking in-line handle can be placed on the diaphragm to expose the hiatus.
- With the stomach retracted toward the left by an assistant through the left upper quadrant port, the gastrohepatic ligament is divided.
- The stomach is then retracted to the right, and the short gastric vessels are divided either with electrocautery or a sealer device (**Fig. 3**). Short gastric mobilization is necessary to achieve a tension-free wrap.
- A retroesophageal window is then created bluntly from the right side with care not to injure the posterior vagus nerve (**Fig. 4**). The right crus should be dissected so that the gastroesophageal junction can be clearly identified and an adequate length of intra-abdominal esophagus is confirmed.
- A posterior crural repair is then performed in all cases to decrease the risk of hiatal hernia formation postoperatively.

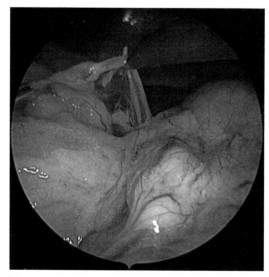

Fig. 3. The stomach is retracted to the right and the short gastric vessels are divided with electrocautery.

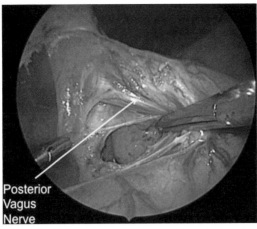

Fig. 4. A retroesophageal window is bluntly created from the right side. Arrow indicates the posterior vagus nerve.

- The stomach is brought through the retroesophageal window and a shoeshine maneuver is performed to assure that the stomach is not twisted.
- The fundoplication wrap is then performed with 3 sutures (**Fig. 5**). The most superior suture incorporates a small piece of anterior esophagus and right crus to help secure the wrap. The 2 more inferior sutures incorporate just anterior esophagus. The wrap should be approximately 2 cm to 3 cm and oriented at the 11-o'clock position. In addition, it is important for the wrap to be above the gastroesophageal junction.

If there is a large defect or recurrent hiatal hernia, the crural repair should be performed with pledgets and horizontal mattress sutures. An orogastric tube is usually

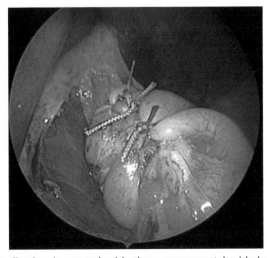

Fig. 5. The fundoplication is created with three permanent braided sutures. The wrap should be approximately 2 cm to 3 cm, floppy, and oriented at the 11-o'clock position.

sufficient to complete the wrap particularly in smaller infants. A bougie may be placed, however, before the fundoplication wrap is performed to avoid creating too tight a wrap around the distal esophagus. Ostlie and colleagues[11] published a table of appropriate bougie sizes for infants weighing less than 15 kg. If a gastrostomy is required, the trocar site in the left upper quadrant is used for the button site. Several techniques may be used to create the gastrostomy, such as securing the stomach to the fascia with laparoscopic sutures and using a wire and sequential dilators to place a button or bringing the stomach to the port site and placing Stamm sutures and a purse-tring suture around the gastrostomy tube.

POSTOPERATIVE CARE

For patients who had a gastrostomy button placed at the time of fundoplication, feeds can usually be started on the first postoperative day and advanced as tolerated. If no gastrostomy was placed, clear liquid diet may be started 4 hours to 6 hours postoperatively.

COMPLICATIONS

Complications after laparoscopic Nissen fundoplication include hiatal hernia, slipped wrap, recurrent GERD, persistent dysphagia, and gas bloat syndrome. Risk factors for recurrence include younger age, preoperative hiatal hernia, postoperative retching, and postoperative esophageal dilation.[12] Postoperative dysphagia may initially be due to swelling of the wrap and subside after the edema has resolved. Occasionally, however, esophageal dilations are required to widen the distal esophagus.

EVIDENCE

Antireflux operations are among the most common procedures performed by pediatric surgeons in the United States. A systematic review of the literature from 1995 to 2010 with 1280 children demonstrated a success rate, as defined as complete relief of reflux symptoms, of 86% in the short term and 72% in the long term.[1] Rothenberg[10] reported his experience with 2000 Nissen fundoplications over 2 decades and found a wrap failure rate of 4.6%. Children with respiratory symptoms, in particular steroid-dependent asthma, seem to have the greatest benefit from antireflux surgery.[13,14]

CONTROVERSIES

The decision for surgical management of GERD is controversial and is often influenced by local and referral cultures. Additionally, pediatric surgeons have differing views on the timing of surgery. Optimal preoperative evaluation allows for better selection of patients and maximization of antireflux surgery. There are also several different operations approaches aside from the Nissen that have been developed for the surgical treatment of GERD, such as partial wraps, which have shown similar outcomes.[15–17]

Several technical aspects during fundoplication have been implicated in increased rates of recurrent GERD and reoperation. Minimal dissection of the esophagus leaving the phrenoesophageal membrane intact has been shown to decrease the incidence of postoperative wrap herniation and the need for reoperation.[18] In addition, crural repair is necessary to minimize hiatal hernia formation and adequate esophageal length is necessary to minimize slippage of the wrap above the hiatus.[19] Finally, some surgeons have shown that crural suturing decreases recurrent GERD.[20] Future studies are necessary to fully evaluate the mechanisms of wrap failure and reasons for recurrence to minimize the relapse of symptoms, complications, and need for reoperation.

There is ongoing controversy regarding the best management for neurologically impaired infants and children with GERD. Some investigators recommend gastrojejunostomies instead of fundoplication in these patients. A meta-analysis comparing these options suggested that there were more major complications with fundoplications and more minor complications with gastrojejunostomies.[21]

SUMMARY

GERD is frequently encountered in infants. Many have resolution of symptoms over time or with nonoperative methods, such as medications. A percentage of patients, however, require surgical treatment due to the persistence of symptoms, ALTEs, poor weight gain, or FTT. There are several tests available for the diagnosis of GERD and for evaluation of the anatomy of the upper gastrointestinal tract. Laparoscopic Nissen fundoplication has become the standard of care for surgical treatment of children with GERD. It has a low morbidity rate and recurrence rates. The key technical points of the operation include creation of an adequate intra-abdominal esophagus, minimal dissection of the hiatus with exposure of the right crus to identify the gastroesophageal junction, crural repair, and creation of floppy, 360° wrap that is oriented at the 11-o'clock position. There are several controversial aspects regarding the management of GERD, including the indications and timing of surgical management, optimal patient selection, and technical modifications to prevent recurrence.

Best Practices

GERD

What is the current practice?

Current practices include
- Diagnostic tests: upper gastrointestinal radiography, pH probe testing, or impedance testing
- Medical treatment: dietary modifications and postural changes, antireflux medications (H_2 blockers and proton pump inhibitors)
- Surgical treatment: failure of medical therapy, failure to thrive, continued respiratory symptoms/ALTE, complications from reflux

Best practice/guideline/care path objective(s)

What changes in current practice are likely to improve outcomes?

- Indications for surgery: better preoperative evaluation/selection of patients (especially for neurologically impaired patients) as well as optimal timing for surgery

- Surgical techniques (Nissen fundoplication): minimal dissection and crural repair

Major recommendations

- Technical recommendations for Nissen: 5 trocars (with one for retraction), division of short gastric vessels to avoid tension of the wrap, dissect right diaphragmatic crus to identify GE junction and obtain adequate intra-abdominal esophageal length, posterior crural repair to reduce the risk of post-operative hiatal hernia formation, floppy wrap placed at the 11-o'clock position, 2 cm to 3 cm in length

Data from Refs.[18–20]

REFERENCES

1. Mauritz FA, van Herwaarden-Lindeboom MY, Stomp W, et al. The effects and efficacy of antireflux surgery in children with gastroesophageal reflux disease: a systematic review. J Gastrointest Surg 2011;15(10):1872–8.
2. Iqbal CW, Holcomb GW 3rd. Gastroesophageal reflux. In: Holcomb GW 3rd, Murphy JP, Ostlie DJ, editors. Ashcraft's pediatric surgery, Vol., 6th edition. London: Elsevier; 2014. p. 387–402.
3. Omari T. Gastro-oesophageal reflux disease in infants and children: new insights, developments and old chestnuts. J Pediatr Gastroenterol Nutr 2005;41(Suppl 1): S21–3.
4. Hollwarth ME. Gastroesophageal reflux disease. In: Coran AG, Adzick NS, Krummel TM, et al, editors. Pediatric surgery, Vol., 7th edition. Philadelphia: Elsevier; 2012. p. 947–58.
5. Wakeman DS, Wilson NA, Warner BW. Current status of surgical management of gastroesophageal reflux in children. Curr Opin Pediatr 2016;28(3):356–62.
6. Mousa HM, Rosen R, Woodley FW, et al. Esophageal impedance monitoring for gastroesophageal reflux. J Pediatr Gastroenterol Nutr 2011;52(2):129–39.
7. Craig WR, Hanlon-Dearman A, Sinclair C, et al. WITHDRAWN: metoclopramide, thickened feedings, and positioning for gastro-oesophageal reflux in children under two years. Cochrane Database Syst Rev 2010;(5):CD003502.
8. Rothenberg SS. The first decade's experience with laparoscopic Nissen fundoplication in infants and children. J Pediatr Surg 2005;40(1):142–6 [discussion: 147].
9. Rothenberg SS. Experience with 220 consecutive laparoscopic Nissen fundoplications in infants and children. J Pediatr Surg Feb 1998;33(2):274–8.
10. Rothenberg SS. Two decades of experience with laparoscopic nissen fundoplication in infants and children: a critical evaluation of indications, technique, and results. J Laparoendosc Adv Surg Tech A 2013;23(9):791–4.
11. Ostlie DJ, Miller KA, Holcomb GW 3rd. Effective Nissen fundoplication length and bougie diameter size in young children undergoing laparoscopic Nissen fundoplication. J Pediatr Surg 2002;37(12):1664–6.
12. Ngerncham M, Barnhart DC, Haricharan RN, et al. Risk factors for recurrent gastroesophageal reflux disease after fundoplication in pediatric patients: a case-control study. J Pediatr Surg 2007;42(9):1478–85.
13. Vandenplas Y, Rudolph CD, Di Lorenzo C, et al. Pediatric gastroesophageal reflux clinical practice guidelines: joint recommendations of the North American Society for Pediatric Gastroenterology, Hepatology, and Nutrition (NASPGHAN) and the European Society for Pediatric Gastroenterology, Hepatology, and Nutrition (ESPGHAN). J Pediatr Gastroenterol Nutr 2009;49(4):498–547.
14. Rothenberg S, Cowles R. The effects of laparoscopic Nissen fundoplication on patients with severe gastroesophageal reflux disease and steroid-dependent asthma. J Pediatr Surg 2012;47(6):1101–4.
15. Esposito C, Montupet P, van Der Zee D, et al. Long-term outcome of laparoscopic Nissen, Toupet, and Thal antireflux procedures for neurologically normal children with gastroesophageal reflux disease. Surg Endosc 2006;20(6):855–8.
16. Kubiak R, Andrews J, Grant HW. Laparoscopic Nissen fundoplication versus Thal fundoplication in children: comparison of short-term outcomes. J Laparoendosc Adv Surg Tech A 2010;20(7):665–9.
17. Kubiak R, Andrews J, Grant HW. Long-term outcome of laparoscopic nissen fundoplication compared with laparoscopic thal fundoplication in children: a prospective, randomized study. Ann Surg 2011;253(1):44–9.

18. Desai AA, Alemayehu H, Holcomb GW 3rd, et al. Minimal vs. maximal esophageal dissection and mobilization during laparoscopic fundoplication: long-term follow-up from a prospective, randomized trial. J Pediatr Surg 2015;50(1):111–4.

19. Bansal S, Rothenberg SS. Evaluation of laparoscopic management of recurrent gastroesophageal reflux disease and hiatal hernia: long term results and evaluation of changing trends. J Pediatr Surg 2014;49(1):72–5 [discussion: 75–6].

20. Hassan ME. Unilateral versus bilateral wrap crural fixation in laparoscopic Nissen fundoplication for children. JSLS 2014;18(4) [pii:e2014.001294].

21. Livingston MH, Shawyer AC, Rosenbaum PL, et al. Fundoplication and gastrostomy versus percutaneous gastrojejunostomy for gastroesophageal reflux in children with neurologic impairment: a systematic review and meta-analysis. J Pediatr Surg 2015;50(5):707–14.

Minimally Invasive Hepatobiliary Surgery

Omid Madadi-Sanjani, MD*, Claus Petersen, PhD, Benno Ure, PhD

KEYWORDS

- Hepatobiliary disease • Laparoscopy • Choledochal cyst excision
- Hepaticoduodenostomy • Hepaticojejunostomy • Kasai procedure
- Cholecystectomy • Hepatic biopsy

KEY POINTS

- Improvements in the available instrumentation and sealing devices, have made pediatric surgeons able to tackle numerous types of demanding procedures laparoscopically.
- Comparative studies and large-scale case series that confirm the advantages of laparoscopy in children with hepatobiliary diseases are scarce.
- Current data indicates that minimally invasive techniques can be recommended for the resection of choledochal cysts and for cholecystectomy.
- More data are required before a recommendation on the use of minimally invasive techniques for biliary atresia and hepatic tumors can be presented.

INTRODUCTION

Two decades ago, surgery for complex biliary conditions in infants and children required an upper abdominal or subcostal incision. In more recent years, as a result of improvements in the instrumentation and sealing devices that are available, pediatric surgeons have been able to tackle numerous types of demanding procedures laparoscopically. These procedures include the resection of choledochal cysts and hepatoportoenterostomy for biliary atresia.

Numerous publications and book chapters have focused on the technical aspects of minimally invasive surgery in infants and children with hepatobiliary diseases. However, comparative studies and large-scale case series that confirm the advantages of laparoscopy in these patients are scarce. As a consequence, there is an ongoing debate as to the advantages and disadvantages of the use of minimally invasive

Disclosure: The authors have no relationship with any commercial company that has direct financial interest in the subject matter or materials discussed in this article or with any organization that manufactures or distributes any products related to this research.
Centre of Pediatric Surgery Hannover, Hannover Medical School, Carl-Neuberg-Street 1, Hannover 30625, Germany
* Corresponding author.
E-mail address: madadi-sanjani.omid@mh-hannover.de

techniques for various biliary conditions and an international consensus on the pros and cons of such surgical approaches has yet to be reached. The discussion has become further complicated following the introduction of single-incision laparoscopic surgery and the use of robotics.

This article presents an overview of the current literature that describes laparoscopic and robotic surgery in pediatric patients with choledochal cyst, biliary atresia, gallbladder diseases, and hepatobiliary malignancies. Comparative studies and case series published in the English language in peer-reviewed journals accessible via PubMed were analyzed. Reports on adult patients were excluded. The evidence levels of the publications that met the inclusion criteria were determined using the Oxford Score.[1]

CHOLEDOCHAL CYST

Choledochal cysts are diagnosed in infancy and childhood either as an incidental ultrasonographical finding or in the course of investigating abdominal symptoms. Occasionally, the diagnosis is established prenatally.[2] The first case report of a child undergoing laparoscopic resection of choledochal cyst and hepaticojejunostomy was published in 1995.[3]

In their systematic review and meta-analysis, Zhen and colleagues[4] recently identified 7 studies that compared children who had undergone laparoscopic choledochal cyst excision (n = 611) with those who had undergone open (n = 797) choledochal cyst excision. The data included in all 7 studies had been collected retrospectively (Oxford evidence-based medicine level IIA). The review confirmed that laparoscopically operated patients underwent a longer operation (7 studies), stayed in hospital for a shorter period (5 studies), and recovered their bowel function faster (3 studies) than those who had undergone open surgery. There were no cases of pancreatitis in laparoscopically operated patients versus 8 such cases following open surgery. The relative risk of intraoperative bleeding was also higher with higher blood transfusion rates in open surgery than laparoscopic (3 studies), but the rate of bile leaks was similar in both groups. Another recent meta-analysis, by Shen and colleagues,[5] which included 1016 patients, confirmed these results. Recently, Yu and colleagues[6] and Ng and colleagues[7] performed comparative studies that showed the safety and feasibility of laparoscopic choledochal cyst excision and they concluded that it had a low complication rate (**Table 1**).

The authors additionally analyzed case studies that examined the use of laparoscopy for choledochal cysts in infants and children that were published on MEDLINE before February 2017. Only series that dealt with children and involved more than 15 patients were included in this review. Seven reports were identified, 6 of which were retrospective (Oxford evidence-based medicine level IIIB) and 1 prospective case series (Oxford evidence-based medicine level IIB). Altogether, 1266 patients were included (**Table 2**).[8–14] These studies confirmed that laparoscopic surgery offers excellent feasibility (see **Table 2**). The conversion rate was 5.2% (16 of 310 procedures). Intraoperative complications were reported in 44 out of 275 patients, and there was no mortality. Furthermore, the mean or median operation time was long and, in 1 study, was more than 7 hours.[6,7]

Note that the level of evidence on the postulated equivalent or better outcomes of laparoscopic versus open surgery is considerably low (Oxford evidence-based medicine level IIIB). Patient and surgeon selection bias cannot be excluded. Therefore, a randomized controlled trial would be required before any general recommendation can be given. In addition, these operations have generally been performed in centers of excellence, and the complication rate associated with general use of the technique remains unclear.

Table 1
Comparative studies on laparoscopic versus open choledochal cyst excision (publications with >15 cases)

Publication	Patient Population (N)	Age (Mean; Lap vs Open)	Operative Time (min; Mean, Lap vs Open)	Hospital Stay (d; Mean, Lap vs Open)	Intraoperative Complications (N; Lap vs Open)	Conversions, N (%)
Yu et al,[6] 2016	156	5.6 vs 5.9 y	—	—	7 vs 8	—
Ng et al,[7] 2014	35	36.5 vs 36.5 mo	536.0 vs 300.0	6.0 vs 5.0	1 vs 5	3 (23.1)
Cherqaoui et al,[76] 2012	19	53.7 vs 62.5 mo	288.6 vs 206.0	12.7 vs 7.9	1 vs 1	0
Liem et al,[77] 2011	616	48.7 vs 63.5 mo	211.0 vs 145.0	7.0 vs 9.1	2 vs 1	2 (0.6)
Diao et al,[78] 2011	418	4.2 vs 4.6 y	195.0 vs 182.4	7.41 vs 9.94	—	—
Liuming et al,[79] 2011	77	5.0 vs 4.0 y	241.0 vs 190	5.5 vs 7.0	1 vs 1	—
She et al,[80] 2009	75	45.0 mo	392 vs 281.0	9.5 vs 6.8	2 vs 3	5 (50)
Aspelund et al,[81] 2007	16	230 vs 234 wk	392	9.5	2 vs 3	0

Abbreviations: lap, laparoscopic choledochal cyst excision; open, open choledochal cyst excision.

Table 2
Case series on laparoscopic choledochal cyst excision (publications with >25 cases)

Publication	Patient Population (N)	Age (Mean)	Operative Time (min; Mean)	Hospital Stay (d; Mean)	Intraoperative Complications (N or %)	Conversions (N or %)
Wen et al,[8] 2017	104	35.9 mo	352.2 (early) vs 240.5 (late)	9.4 (early) vs 7.8 (late)	13.5% (early) vs 1.5% (late)	10.8% (early) vs 4.5% (late)
Qiao et al,[9] 2015	956	4.01 y	211.2	—	—	—
Wang et al,[10] 2012	41	4.0 y	210	7.2	16	1
Tang et al,[11] 2011	62	2.3 y	226	8.0	8.2%	1.6%
Lee et al,[12] 2009	37	4.3 y	439	—	13	3
Hong et al,[13] 2008	31	45.2 mo	312	8.6	4	4
Li et al,[14] 2004	35	3.6 y	258	4.5	—	0

Abbreviations: Early, early experiences in lap; late, late experiences in lap.

Several other aspects of laparoscopic choledochal cyst excision have been investigated. Hepaticojejunostomy is currently the preferred technique. It was recently postulated that hepaticoduodenostomy would be technically easier and is associated with a shorter mean operative time, less intraoperative blood loss, and equivalent intraoperative complication rates.[15–17] However, initial reports have to be treated carefully. The authors identified 6 studies on laparoscopic hepaticoduodenostomy versus hepaticojejunostomy that had inconclusive results.[15,17–21] Santore and colleagues[19] reported a lower complication rate in 39 patients after hepaticoduodenostomy compared with 20 after hepaticojejunostomy; however, the rate of complications after jejunostomy was 20% and, as such, was unacceptably high (Oxford evidence-based medicine level IIIB). In one review, Narayanan and colleagues[22] analyzed the results of 6 retrospective studies that compared patients who underwent open or laparoscopic hepaticojejunostomy (n = 267) and hepaticoduodenostomy (n = 412). The investigators concluded that the data showed equivalent results in postoperative bile leak and anastomotic stricture, whereas rates of cholangitis and bile reflux were higher after hepaticoduodenostomy (Oxford evidence-based medicine level IIA).

Three studies on single-incision laparoscopic cyst excision were identified.[23–25] The results relating to operation duration, intraoperative complications, conversion rates, and length of hospital stay were comparable with those related to conventional laparoscopic cyst excision reported in the literature.

Information on the feasibility of the use of laparoscopic treatment with forme fruste choledochal cysts is scarce. Kirschner and colleagues[26] reported the use of the procedure with 7 children with 1 conversion. One child had an anastomotic leak.

Martino and colleagues[27] presented a case of postoperative gastrointestinal bleeding following laparoscopic treatment of forme fruste choledochal cyst; however, they concluded that this was not associated with the operation.

Total laparoscopic management includes an intracorporeal hepaticojejunostomy. Urushihara and colleagues[28] reported good feasibility without conversion and a mean operative time of 390 minutes in 8 children. Ahn and colleagues[29] documented 38 minutes for the intracorporeal anastomosis. Gander and colleagues[30] hypothesized that a potential benefit of this technique is that it involves minimal handling of the bowel, which could minimize postoperative ileus. Their median operative time was 240 minutes with initiation of diet on postoperative day 1. Lee and colleagues[31] reported reoperation of a bowel stricture in a patient at the 7-month follow-up.

Diao and colleagues[32] investigated whether an intraoperative placement of a drain is necessary in the laparoscopic era. A prospective, randomized study including 100 children was performed (Oxford evidence-based medicine level IB). The intensity of pain was significantly higher in the drainage group. Furthermore, the resumption of normal activity was faster, and the duration of postoperative hospital stay shorter in patients without drainage.

In 2010, Dawrant and colleagues[33] reported a robot-assisted resection of choledochal cyst. The mean operating time was 8 hours and diet was initiated after a median of 3 days following operation. The same group could not successfully reduce the operative time in another 22 cases that were subsequently operated on.[34]

In addition, the incidence of cancer in adult patients with choledochal cyst has been reported to be up to 11%.[35] In addition, there also remains a long-term risk of cancer after operation, and this risk has been reported to be higher in incompletely resected cysts. Long-term results after laparoscopic resection of choledochal cyst are not yet available. Systematic lifelong follow-up remains mandatory in all patients with choledochal cyst, regardless of which form of operation they have undergone.

KASAI PORTOENTEROSTOMY

Biliary atresia represents the leading cause of death from liver failure and the most frequent indication for liver transplant in infants and children.[36,37] The outcome depends on timely performance of Kasai portoenterostomy.[38] The objective of the portoenterostomy is to restore bile drainage, which can be achieved in about 50% of the patients in the short-term. However, long-term deterioration of the liver function occurs in up to 80% of all patients with biliary atresia who eventually require liver transplant.[39,40] The postoperative outcome measures after Kasai portoenterostomy are overall survival, survival with native liver, and jaundice-free survival with native liver.

The primary objective of performing Kasai procedures using minimally invasive techniques was to reduce surgical trauma and postoperative pain, and to ease liver explantation when liver transplant became necessary. However, many experts raised concerns about the use of this technique and, during a panel discussion that was held at the annual meeting of the International Pediatric Endosurgical Group in 2007, 4 of 5 surgeons stated that they had stopped using laparoscopy for patients with biliary atresia.

A recent review and meta-analysis (Oxford evidence-based medicine level IIA) included 9 retrospective and 2 prospective studies that compared laparoscopic and open Kasai portoenterostomy.[41] The analysis confirmed that, in most of the studies, patients who underwent laparoscopic surgery endured a longer operation time and a significantly lower rate of 2-year survival with native liver than those who underwent conventional Kasai. Hospital stay, early clearance of jaundice, and the incidence of cholangitis were not significantly different. The investigators concluded that laparoscopy could not be recommended for infants with biliary atresia. Hussain and colleagues[42] also published a review that included 10 studies with 148 patients (Oxford evidence-based medicine level IIA). They confirmed the conclusion mentioned earlier.

The authors analyzed all studies on laparoscopic Kasai portoenterostomy in the English language that included 20 or more patients (**Table 3**). The first prospective trial comparing laparoscopic and conventional Kasai portoenterostomy in a high-caseload European institution had to be stopped for ethical reasons.[43] Interim analysis revealed lower rates of jaundice-free survival with native liver and survival with native liver as well as a high rate of liver failure and early transplant after laparoscopic surgery (Oxford evidence-based medicine level IIB). Poor results after laparoscopic Kasai were also reported by Chan and colleagues.[44,45] Furthermore, Oetzmann von Sochaczewski and colleagues[46] could not confirm faster liver explantation in cases with liver transplant because of fewer abdominal adhesions after minimally invasive Kasai procedures (Oxford evidence-based medicine level IIIB). However, a recent prospective randomized trial conducted by Sun and colleagues[47] included 91 patients and found that the short-term and midterm results were comparable for both groups (Oxford evidence-based medicine level IB).

Revision of Kasai portoenterostomy has been suggested for patients with jaundice recurrence and recurrent cholangitis.[48,49] Murase and colleagues[50] reported on successful laparoscopic revision of an initial laparoscopic Kasai procedure. There were no conversions or intraoperative complications, and 3 children survived with native liver.

Reports on robotic-assisted Kasai portoenterostomy are scarce. An initial case series on the use of the Da Vinci system included 3 children.[51] The investigators emphasized the high definition of Da Vinci endoscopes. No information on the duration of operation and setup were given. Meehan and colleagues[52] reported on 2 patients who underwent operations that were conducted according to the Da Vinci system.

Table 3
Studies on laparoscopic and laparoscopic versus open Kasai portoenterostomy (publications with >20 cases)

Publication	Techniques	Patient Population (N)	Age, Lap vs Open (d. Mean)	Operative Time, Lap vs Open (min, Mean)	Jaundice-free SNL[a] Follow-up, Lap vs Open (mo); N (%)	SNL Follow-up, Lap vs Open (mo); N (%)	LTx Follow-up, Lap vs Open (mo); N (%)	Complications (N)	Summary
Sun et al,[47] 2016	Lap vs open	91	61.5 vs 67.0	169.5 vs 146.0	—	36 (82%) vs 40 (85%) (6 mo)	—	—	No significant differences in short-term and midterm results
Nakamura et al,[82] 2016	Lap vs open	31	65.5 vs 69.3	—	—	13 (76.5%) vs 10 (71.4%) (2.5 y)	4 (23.5%) vs 4 (28.6%) (2.5 y)	—	Jaundice-clearance rate better in lap group
Chan et al,[44] 2014	Lap vs open	43	65.6 vs 58.9	—	8 (50%) vs 22 (81%) (6 mo)	8 (50%) vs 22 (81%) (2 y)	—	—	Open surgery is associated with superior JF-SNL and 2-y SNL
Wang et al,[83] 2014	Lap	25	72.0	208	12 (48%) (3-24 mo)	—	—	0	Laparoscopic technique is safe and feasible
Wada et al,[84] 2014	Lap vs open	23	65.8 vs 64.7	546 vs 468	—	9 (75%) vs 9 (82%) (2 y)	3 (25%) vs 2 (18%) (2 y)	—	Lap Kasai cannot replace open Kasai; open Kasai remains gold standard
Ure et al,[43] 2011	Lap vs open	41	57.0 vs 57.0	—	2 (17%) vs 11 (39%) (6 mo)	5 (42%) vs 23 (82%) (6 mo)	10 (83%) vs 18 (64%) (24 mo)	0	Lower SNL in laparoscopy group; lap is technically feasible
Martinez-Ferro et al,[85] 2005[b]	Lap	41	43.0 (A) and 79.1 (B)	150.0 (A) 210.0 (B)	—	—	16 (39.0%) (13 mo)	3	Laparoscopy is feasible; encouraging results

Abbreviations: lap, laparoscopic Kasai portoenterostomy; LTx, liver transplant rate; open, open Kasai portoenterostomy; SNL, survival with native liver.
[a] Direct serum bilirubin level less than 20 μL/mol/L.
[b] Two locations (A and B).

There were no perioperative complications, but the duration of the operation was longer than 6 hours.

The authors conclude that more studies with higher patient numbers are mandatory before laparoscopic Kasai portoenterostomy can be recommended.

CHOLECYSTECTOMY

When reviewing the literature of laparoscopic biliary surgery in children, it becomes apparent that most reports deal with cholecystectomy. The operation is recommended for children with symptomatic gallstone disease and for (asymptomatic) patients with hemolytic diseases such as sickle cell disease.[53] More recently, biliary dyskinesia has been introduced as an indication for cholecystectomy.[54]

In a recent review, Dagash and colleagues[55] included 11 studies and 20,246 patients who had undergone laparoscopic cholecystectomy (Oxford evidence-based medicine level IIA). The feasibility was excellent after a substantial learning curve with a decrease in operation duration, conversion rate, and postoperative hospital stay during the observational periods. In his review, Davenport[56] emphasized that the postoperative recovery time and hospital time had reduced and better cosmesis had been observed in children following laparoscopic cholecystectomy than in those treated by open surgery. However, difficulties with intraoperative cholangiography in cases with choledocholithiasis limited the feasibility of the study (Oxford evidence-based medicine level IIIA), and this was confirmed in a further review by Zitsman.[57]

Campbell and colleagues[58] reported on 16 children who underwent laparoscopic cholecystectomy for biliary dyskinesia with a success rate of 94%. Other investigators achieved a resolution of symptoms in 77%[59] and 76%[60] of cases (Oxford evidence-based medicine level IIIB). Lacher and colleagues[61] and Lyons and colleagues[62] confirmed a good postoperative outcomes, in particular in patients with a low ejection fraction in cholescintigraphy (Oxford evidence-based medicine level IIIB).

However, Scott Nelson and colleagues[63] showed equal symptom resolution in conservatively and operatively treated children after 2 years of follow-up (Oxford evidence-based medicine level IIIB).

In their review on single-incision cholecystectomy, Chrestiana and colleagues[64] concluded that single-incision laparoscopic surgery is feasible and safe but technically challenging. Holcomb[65] summarized the results of a pediatric case series on single-incision cholecystectomy and found low complication and conversion rates with comparable operation duration compared with conventional laparoscopy (Oxford evidence-based medicine level IIA). Another review confirmed similar operating time, morbidity, and intensity of pain when comparing single-incision and multiport laparoscopic cholecystectomy (Oxford evidence-based medicine level IIA).[66] However, in their randomized trial, Ostlie and colleagues[67] enrolled 60 patients and identified a longer operative time, a greater degree of difficulty, more doses of analgesics used, and greater hospital charges in the single-site group, which trended toward significance (Oxford evidence-based medicine level IB).

Several preliminary reports on robotic-assisted cholecystectomy in children are available. A median operative time of 125 minutes and a median duration of operation of 77 minutes in 14 patients was reported by Rosales-Velderrain and colleagues.[68] There were no conversions and no complications besides a port site seroma (Oxford evidence-based medicine level IIIB).

Similar outcomes were confirmed by Jones[69] in a series that investigated cases involving 16 children. However, because of the higher cost of the surgery and lack of solid evidence as to its advantages, the use of robotics for cholecystectomy cannot yet be recommended.[70]

HEPATIC TUMORS

Information on minimally invasive surgery for pediatric hepatobiliary tumors is scarce. Kim and colleagues[71] reported on 2 laparoscopic partial hepatectomies for hepatoblastoma. Both resected tumors were small (3.5 and 2.5 cm maximum in diameter) and were located in easily accessible segments 5 and 6. The operations were feasible but required a team experienced in minimally invasive as well as liver surgery. Yada and colleagues[72] subsequently reported on another case of a patient who underwent laparoscopic hepatoblastoma resection over a total operation time of 225 minutes. The investigators emphasized the benefits of magnification leading to a better visual field compared with open surgery (Oxford evidence-based medicine level V). It may be concluded that the reported data on the use of minimally invasive surgery for resection of hepatobiliary tumors are scarce and, therefore, more experience is required before a general recommendation can be presented.

An excellent feasibility of laparoscopic biopsies for pediatric hepatobiliary tumors was reported by several investigators.[73–75] In these series, most cases involved liver tumors, which were mainly hepatoblastoma. The investigators described the technique as simple with a low complication rate and an excellent diagnostic accuracy (Oxford evidence-based medicine level IIIB).

SUMMARY

Comparative studies and large case series that confirm the advantages of laparoscopy to operate on most hepatobiliary diseases in children remain scarce. The level of evidence to support the use of minimally invasive techniques in these patients remains low. The review presented in this article indicates that minimally invasive techniques can be recommended for the resection of choledochal cysts and for cholecystectomy. More data are required before a recommendation on the use of minimally invasive techniques for other hepatobiliary conditions, such as biliary atresia or tumors, can be presented.

Best Practices

Minimal invasive hepatobiliary surgery in children

What is the current practice?

Best practice/guideline/care path objectives
- Early referral to centers of excellence specializing in pediatric surgery and hepatology
- Selection of children for laparoscopy based on disease, age, equipment, and experience
- Based on these criteria: laparoscopic choledochal cyst excision, open Kasai portoenterostomy and single-incision or 3-port laparoscopic cholecystectomy

What changes in current practice are likely to improve outcomes?

- Introduction of screening methods for early detection of hepatobiliary diseases

- Centralization, with referral of children to pediatric centers specializing in hepatobiliary disorders

- Further development of laparoscopic and robotic equipment for pediatric patients

- International registries, especially for biliary atresia, for exchange of treatment and follow-up data and therefore the improvement of care

Major recommendations

- Laparoscopic choledochal cyst excision can be considered in most pediatric patients under supervision of an experienced pediatric surgeon if specialized equipment is available (grade 3B)
- Open Kasai portoenterostomy at centers with intensive interdisciplinary cooperation of pediatric surgeons, hepatologists, and transplant surgeons should be preferred because of the superior long-term outcomes (grade 2A)
- Single-incision and 3-port laparoscopic cholecystectomy should be the treatment of choice in children (grade 2A)
- There is no evidence for the use of laparoscopy in hepatic tumor surgery

Summary statement

The level of evidence for the use of minimally invasive techniques in children with hepatobiliary disorders remains low. Current data indicate that minimally invasive techniques can be recommended for the resection of choledochal cysts and for cholecystectomy.

REFERENCES

1. Oxford Centre for Evidence-based Medicine - Levels of Evidence (March 2009). CEBM. 2009. Available at: http://www.cebm.net/oxford-centre-evidence-based-medicine-levels-evidence-march-2009/. Accessed April 7, 2017.
2. Weng R, Hu W, Cai S, et al. Prenatal diagnosis and prognosis assessment of congenital choledochal cyst in 21 cases. J Obstet Gynaecol 2016;36(3):324–7.
3. Farello GA, Cerofolini A, Rebonato M, et al. Congenital choledochal cyst: video-guided laparoscopic treatment. Surg Laparosc Endosc 1995;5(5):354–8.
4. Zhen C, Xia Z, Long L, et al. Laparoscopic excision versus open excision for the treatment of choledochal cysts: a systematic review and meta-analysis. Int Surg 2015;100(1):115–22.
5. Shen H-J, Xu M, Zhu H-Y, et al. Laparoscopic versus open surgery in children with choledochal cysts: a meta-analysis. Pediatr Surg Int 2015;31(6):529–34.
6. Yu B-H, Lin F. Clinical effects in resection of congenital choledochal cyst of children and jejunum Roux-Y anastomosis by laparoscope. Eur Rev Med Pharmacol Sci 2016;20(21):4530–4.
7. Ng JL, Salim MT, Low Y. Mid-term outcomes of laparoscopic versus open choledochal cyst excision in a tertiary paediatric hospital. Ann Acad Med Singapore 2014;43(4):220–4.
8. Wen Z, Liang H, Liang J, et al. Evaluation of the learning curve of laparoscopic choledochal cyst excision and Roux-en-Y hepaticojejunostomy in children: CUSUM analysis of a single surgeon's experience. Surg Endosc 2017;31(2):778–87.
9. Qiao G, Li L, Li S, et al. Laparoscopic cyst excision and Roux-Y hepaticojejunostomy for children with choledochal cysts in China: a multicenter study. Surg Endosc 2015;29(1):140–4.
10. Wang B, Feng Q, Mao J, et al. Early experience with laparoscopic excision of choledochal cyst in 41 children. J Pediatr Surg 2012;47(12):2175–8.
11. Tang S-T, Yang Y, Wang Y, et al. Laparoscopic choledochal cyst excision, hepaticojejunostomy, and extracorporeal Roux-en-Y anastomosis: a technical skill and intermediate-term report in 62 cases. Surg Endosc 2011;25(2):416–22.
12. Lee KH, Tam YH, Yeung CK, et al. Laparoscopic excision of choledochal cysts in children: an intermediate-term report. Pediatr Surg Int 2009;25(4):355–60.

13. Hong L, Wu Y, Yan Z, et al. Laparoscopic surgery for choledochal cyst in children: a case review of 31 patients. Eur J Pediatr Surg 2008;18(2):67–71.
14. Li L, Feng W, Jing-Bo F, et al. Laparoscopic-assisted total cyst excision of choledochal cyst and Roux-en-Y hepatoenterostomy. J Pediatr Surg 2004;39(11): 1663–6.
15. Yeung F, Chung PHY, Wong KKY, et al. Biliary-enteric reconstruction with hepaticoduodenostomy following laparoscopic excision of choledochal cyst is associated with better postoperative outcomes: a single-centre experience. Pediatr Surg Int 2015;31(2):149–53.
16. Liem NT, Dung LA, Son TN. Laparoscopic complete cyst excision and hepaticoduodenostomy for choledochal cyst: early results in 74 cases. J Laparoendosc Adv Surg Tech A 2009;19(Suppl 1):S87–90.
17. Dalton BGA, Gonzalez KW, Dehmer JJ, et al. Transition of techniques to treat choledochal cysts in children. J Laparoendosc Adv Surg Tech A 2016;26(1): 62–5.
18. Senthilnathan P, Patel ND, Nair AS, et al. Laparoscopic management of choledochal cyst-technical modifications and outcome analysis. World J Surg 2015; 39(10):2550–6.
19. Santore MT, Deans KJ, Behar BJ, et al. Laparoscopic hepaticoduodenostomy versus open hepaticoduodenostomy for reconstruction after resection of choledochal cyst. J Laparoendosc Adv Surg Tech A 2011;21(4):375–8.
20. Nguyen Thanh L, Hien PD, Dung LA, et al. Laparoscopic repair for choledochal cyst: lessons learned from 190 cases. J Pediatr Surg 2010;45(3):540–4.
21. Liem NT, Pham HD, Dung LA, et al. Early and intermediate outcomes of laparoscopic surgery for choledochal cysts with 400 patients. J Laparoendosc Adv Surg Tech A 2012;22(6):599–603.
22. Narayanan SK, Chen Y, Narasimhan KL, et al. Hepaticoduodenostomy versus hepaticojejunostomy after resection of choledochal cyst: a systematic review and meta-analysis. J Pediatr Surg 2013;48(11):2336–42.
23. Tang Y, Li F, He G. Comparison of single-incision and conventional laparoscopic cyst excision and Roux-en-Y hepaticojejunostomy for children with choledochal cysts. Indian J Surg 2016;78(4):259–64.
24. Son TN, Liem NT, Hoan VX. Transumbilical laparoendoscopic single-site surgery with conventional instruments for choledochal cyst in children: early results of 86 cases. J Laparoendosc Adv Surg Tech A 2014;24(12):907–10.
25. Diao M, Li L, Cheng W. Single-incision laparoscopic hepaticojejunostomy using conventional instruments for neonates with extrahepatic biliary cystic lesions. Surg Innov 2013;20(3):214–8.
26. Kirschner HJ, Szavay PO, Schaefer JF, et al. Laparoscopic Roux-en-Y hepaticojejunostomy in children with long common pancreaticobiliary channel: surgical technique and functional outcome. J Laparoendosc Adv Surg Tech A 2010; 20(5):485–8.
27. Martino A, Noviello C, Cobellis G, et al. Delayed upper gastrointestinal bleeding after laparoscopic treatment of forme fruste choledochal cyst. J Laparoendosc Adv Surg Tech A 2009;19(3):457–9.
28. Urushihara N, Fukuzawa H, Fukumoto K, et al. Totally laparoscopic management of choledochal cyst: Roux-en-Y jejunojejunostomy and wide hepaticojejunostomy with hilar ductoplasty. J Laparoendosc Adv Surg Tech A 2011;21(4):361–6.
29. Ahn SM, Jun JY, Lee WJ, et al. Laparoscopic total intracorporeal correction of choledochal cyst in pediatric population. J Laparoendosc Adv Surg Tech A 2009;19(5):683–6.

30. Gander JW, Cowles RA, Gross ER, et al. Laparoscopic excision of choledochal cysts with total intracorporeal reconstruction. J Laparoendosc Adv Surg Tech A 2010;20(10):877–81.

31. Lee JS, Yoon YC. Laparoscopic treatment of choledochal cyst using barbed sutures. J Laparoendosc Adv Surg Tech A 2017;27(1):58–62.

32. Diao M, Li L, Cheng W. To drain or not to drain in Roux-en-Y hepatojejunostomy for children with choledochal cysts in the laparoscopic era: a prospective randomized study. J Pediatr Surg 2012;47(8):1485–9.

33. Dawrant MJ, Najmaldin AS, Alizai NK. Robot-assisted resection of choledochal cysts and hepaticojejunostomy in children less than 10 kg. J Pediatr Surg 2010;45(12):2364–8.

34. Alizai NK, Dawrant MJ, Najmaldin AS. Robot-assisted resection of choledochal cysts and hepaticojejunostomy in children. Pediatr Surg Int 2014;30(3):291–4.

35. Ohashi T, Wakai T, Kubota M, et al. Risk of subsequent biliary malignancy in patients undergoing cyst excision for congenital choledochal cysts. J Gastroenterol Hepatol 2013;28(2):243–7.

36. Petersen C, Davenport M. Aetiology of biliary atresia: what is actually known? Orphanet J Rare Dis 2013;8:128.

37. Verkade HJ, Bezerra JA, Davenport M, et al. Biliary atresia and other cholestatic childhood diseases: advances and future challenges. J Hepatol 2016;65(3): 631–42.

38. Nio M, Wada M, Sasaki H, et al. Effects of age at Kasai portoenterostomy on the surgical outcome: a review of the literature. Surg Today 2015;45(7):813–8.

39. Davenport M, Ong E, Sharif K, et al. Biliary atresia in England and Wales: results of centralization and new benchmark. J Pediatr Surg 2011;46(9):1689–94.

40. Chardot C, Buet C, Serinet M-O, et al. Improving outcomes of biliary atresia: French national series 1986-2009. J Hepatol 2013;58(6):1209–17.

41. Lishuang M, Zhen C, Guoliang Q, et al. Laparoscopic portoenterostomy versus open portoenterostomy for the treatment of biliary atresia: a systematic review and meta-analysis of comparative studies. Pediatr Surg Int 2015;31(3):261–9.

42. Hussain MH, Alizai N, Patel B. Outcomes of laparoscopic Kasai portoenterostomy for biliary atresia: a systematic review. J Pediatr Surg 2017;52(2):264–7.

43. Ure BM, Kuebler JF, Schukfeh N, et al. Survival with the native liver after laparoscopic versus conventional Kasai portoenterostomy in infants with biliary atresia: a prospective trial. Ann Surg 2011;253(4):826–30.

44. Chan KWE, Lee KH, Wong HYV, et al. From laparoscopic to open Kasai portoenterostomy: the outcome after reintroduction of open Kasai portoenterostomy in infant with biliary atresia. Pediatr Surg Int 2014;30(6):605–8.

45. Chan KWE, Lee KH, Tsui SYB, et al. Laparoscopic versus open Kasai portoenterostomy in infant with biliary atresia: a retrospective review on the 5-year native liver survival. Pediatr Surg Int 2012;28(11):1109–13.

46. Oetzmann von Sochaczewski C, Petersen C, Ure BM, et al. Laparoscopic versus conventional Kasai portoenterostomy does not facilitate subsequent liver transplantation in infants with biliary atresia. J Laparoendosc Adv Surg Tech A 2012;22(4):408–11.

47. Sun X, Diao M, Wu X, et al. A prospective study comparing laparoscopic and conventional Kasai portoenterostomy in children with biliary atresia. J Pediatr Surg 2016;51(3):374–8.

48. Bondoc AJ, Taylor JA, Alonso MH, et al. The beneficial impact of revision of Kasai portoenterostomy for biliary atresia: an institutional study. Ann Surg 2012;255(3): 570–6.

49. Shirota C, Uchida H, Ono Y, et al. Long-term outcomes after revision of Kasai portoenterostomy for biliary atresia. J Hepatobiliary Pancreat Sci 2016;23(11): 715–20.

50. Murase N, Uchida H, Ono Y, et al. A new era of laparoscopic revision of Kasai portoenterostomy for the treatment of biliary atresia. Biomed Res Int 2015; 2015:173014.

51. Dutta S, Woo R, Albanese CT. Minimal access portoenterostomy: advantages and disadvantages of standard laparoscopic and robotic techniques. J Laparoendosc Adv Surg Tech A 2007;17(2):258–64.

52. Meehan JJ, Elliott S, Sandler A. The robotic approach to complex hepatobiliary anomalies in children: preliminary report. J Pediatr Surg 2007;42(12):2110–4.

53. Svensson J, Makin E. Gallstone disease in children. Semin Pediatr Surg 2012; 21(3):255–65.

54. Halata MS, Berezin SH. Biliary dyskinesia in the pediatric patient. Curr Gastroenterol Rep 2008;10(3):332–8.

55. Dagash H, Chowdhury M, Pierro A. When can I be proficient in laparoscopic surgery? A systematic review of the evidence. J Pediatr Surg 2003;38(5):720–4.

56. Davenport M. Laparoscopic surgery in children. Ann R Coll Surg Engl 2003;85(5): 324–30.

57. Zitsman JL. Current concepts in minimal access surgery for children. Pediatrics 2003;111(6 Pt 1):1239–52.

58. Campbell BT, Narasimhan NP, Golladay ES, et al. Biliary dyskinesia: a potentially unrecognized cause of abdominal pain in children. Pediatr Surg Int 2004;20(8): 579–81.

59. Kaye AJ, Jatla M, Mattei P, et al. Use of laparoscopic cholecystectomy for biliary dyskinesia in the child. J Pediatr Surg 2008;43(6):1057–9.

60. Knott EM, Fike FB, Gasior AC, et al. Multi-institutional analysis of long-term symptom resolution after cholecystectomy for biliary dyskinesia in children. Pediatr Surg Int 2013;29(12):1243–7.

61. Lacher M, Yannam GR, Muensterer OJ, et al. Laparoscopic cholecystectomy for biliary dyskinesia in children: frequency increasing. J Pediatr Surg 2013;48(8): 1716–21.

62. Lyons H, Hagglund KH, Smadi Y. Outcomes after laparoscopic cholecystectomy in children with biliary dyskinesia. Surg Laparosc Endosc Percutan Tech 2011; 21(3):175–8.

63. Scott Nelson R, Kolts R, Park R, et al. A comparison of cholecystectomy and observation in children with biliary dyskinesia. J Pediatr Surg 2006;41(11): 1894–8.

64. Chrestiana D, Sucandy I. Current state of single-port laparoscopic cholecystectomy in children. Am Surg 2013;79(9):897–8.

65. Holcomb GW. Single-site umbilical laparoscopic cholecystectomy. Semin Pediatr Surg 2011;20(4):201–7.

66. Garey CL, Laituri CA, Ostlie DJ, et al. Single-incision laparoscopic surgery in children: initial single-center experience. J Pediatr Surg 2011;46(5):904–7.

67. Ostlie DJ, Juang OOAD, Iqbal CW, et al. Single incision versus standard 4-port laparoscopic cholecystectomy: a prospective randomized trial. J Pediatr Surg 2013;48(1):209–14.

68. Rosales-Velderrain A, Alkhoury F. Single-port robotic cholecystectomy in pediatric patients: single institution experience. J Laparoendosc Adv Surg Tech A 2017; 27(4):434–7.

69. Jones VS. Robotic-assisted single-site cholecystectomy in children. J Pediatr Surg 2015;50(11):1842–5.
70. Mahida JB, Cooper JN, Herz D, et al. Utilization and costs associated with robotic surgery in children. J Surg Res 2015;199(1):169–76.
71. Kim T, Kim D-Y, Cho MJ, et al. Use of laparoscopic surgical resection for pediatric malignant solid tumors: a case series. Surg Endosc 2011;25(5):1484–8.
72. Yada K, Ishibashi H, Mori H, et al. Laparoscopic resection of hepatoblastoma: report of a case. Asian J Endosc Surg 2014;7(3):267–70.
73. Drăghici IM, Luca D-C, Popescu M-D, et al. Technological update of the video-endoscopic approach of the diagnosis and staging of tumors in children. Rom J Morphol Embryol 2014;55(2 Suppl):597–602.
74. Metzelder ML, Kuebler JF, Shimotakahara A, et al. Role of diagnostic and ablative minimally invasive surgery for pediatric malignancies. Cancer 2007;109(11): 2343–8.
75. Holcomb GW, Tomita SS, Haase GM, et al. Minimally invasive surgery in children with cancer. Cancer 1995;76(1):121–8.
76. Cherqaoui A, Haddad M, Roman C, et al. Management of choledochal cyst: evolution with antenatal diagnosis and laparoscopic approach. J Minim Access Surg 2012;8(4):129–33.
77. Liem NT, Pham HD, Vu HM. Is the laparoscopic operation as safe as open operation for choledochal cyst in children? J Laparoendosc Adv Surg Tech A 2011; 21(4):367–70.
78. Diao M, Li L, Cheng W. Laparoscopic versus open Roux-en-Y hepatojejunostomy for children with choledochal cysts: intermediate-term follow-up results. Surg Endosc 2011;25(5):1567–73.
79. Liuming H, Hongwu Z, Gang L, et al. The effect of laparoscopic excision vs open excision in children with choledochal cyst: a midterm follow-up study. J Pediatr Surg 2011;46(4):662–5.
80. She W-H, Chung HY, Lan LCL, et al. Management of choledochal cyst: 30 years of experience and results in a single center. J Pediatr Surg 2009;44(12):2307–11.
81. Aspelund G, Ling SC, Ng V, et al. A role for laparoscopic approach in the treatment of biliary atresia and choledochal cysts. J Pediatr Surg 2007;42(5):869–72.
82. Nakamura H, Koga H, Cazares J, et al. Comprehensive assessment of prognosis after laparoscopic portoenterostomy for biliary atresia. Pediatr Surg Int 2016; 32(2):109–12.
83. Wang B, Feng Q, Ye X, et al. The experience and technique in laparoscopic portoenterostomy for biliary atresia. J Laparoendosc Adv Surg Tech A 2014;24(5): 350–3.
84. Wada M, Nakamura H, Koga H, et al. Experience of treating biliary atresia with three types of portoenterostomy at a single institution: extended, modified Kasai, and laparoscopic modified Kasai. Pediatr Surg Int 2014;30(9):863–70.
85. Martinez-Ferro M, Esteves E, Laje P. Laparoscopic treatment of biliary atresia and choledochal cyst. Semin Pediatr Surg 2005;14(4):206–15.

Minimally Invasive Surgery in the Management of Anorectal Malformations

Sarah B. Cairo, MD, MPH[a], David H. Rothstein, MD, MS[a,b],
Carroll M. Harmon, MD, PhD[a,b],*

KEYWORDS

- Imperforate anus • Anorectal malformation (ARM)
- Posterior sagittal anorectoplasty (PSARP)
- Laparoscopic-assisted anorectal pull-through (LAARP) • Minimally invasive surgery
- Congenital anomalies

KEY POINTS

- Anorectal malformations (ARMs) are common and often associated with other congenital anomalies. There are several different configurations of ARM seen in the neonatal population, with incidence often varying with the presence of associated anomalies.
- The type of repair performed, including laparoscopic-assisted anorectal pull-through and posterior sagittal anorectoplasty, largely depends on surgeon preference, experience, and type of anomaly.
- Further research is needed on long-term functional outcomes of laparoscopic-assisted versus traditional repair of ARM because results may be attributed to the type of ARM and location of the fistula more than the surgical technique.

INTRODUCTION

Imperforate anus, a variant of anorectal malformation (ARM), has been well documented in the medical literature since antiquity, when a variety of crude techniques were used to create an orifice in the perineum.[1] ARM occurs in 1 out of every 4000 to 5000 newborns, with a slightly higher rate among boys.[2] Most ARMs result in absent or abnormal anal orifice and are associated with rectourethral or perineal fistula. A small group of patients have a blind-ending pouch (rectal atresia) without fistula.[3,4] The type of ARM and associated genitourinary anomalies vary with gender such that the most frequently reported ARM in male patients is imperforate anus with a rectourethral fistula. In female patients, rectovestibular fistula and perineal fistulas are reported most

[a] Department of Pediatric Surgery, Women and Children's Hospital of Buffalo, 219 Bryant Street, Buffalo, NY 14222, USA; [b] Department of Surgery, State University of New York, University at Buffalo, 3435 Main Street, Buffalo, NY 14214, USA
* Corresponding author. Women and Children's Hospital, 219 Bryant Street, Buffalo, NY 14222.
E-mail address: carrollh@buffalo.edu

Clin Perinatol 44 (2017) 819–834
http://dx.doi.org/10.1016/j.clp.2017.08.007   **perinatology.theclinics.com**

commonly.[5] Imperforate anus without a fistula accounts for only approximately 5% of all ARMs and is most likely to be associated with Down syndrome.[6] Historically ARMs, and specifically imperforate anus, were described as low, intermediate, or high, in an attempt to describe the space between the supralevator muscle complex and the distal rectum (**Table 1**). This classification was used to guide therapy, whereas traditional perineal approaches were applied to low and occasionally intermediate defects. In contrast, abdominal approaches are often required for high or unknown defects. Of note, there is a higher incidence of associated vertebral, spinal, and genitourinary anomalies in patients with a very high defect compared with lower ones.[7,8]

Compared with other congenital intestinal anomalies, ARM is more often associated with other anomalies, which seems to influence the type of defect and work-up performed. In particular, ARM may be present in up to 90% of patients with the VACTERL (vertebral anomalies, anal atresia, cardiac malformations, tracheoesophageal fistula with or without esophageal atresia, renal dysplasia, and limb [often radial] anomalies) association.[2,5] VACTERL, a nonrandom co-occurrence of congenital malformations affecting between 1 in 10,000 and 1 in 40,000 live births, includes 3 component features and the absence of an encompassing diagnosis.[9,10] In particular, vertebral anomalies are the most frequently associated defect with ARMs with the severity of spinal or vertebral anomaly often correlating with overall prognosis.[11] Regardless of spinal deformity, ARMs present a unique management dilemma based on the wide variety of presentations and frequently associated genitourinary anomalies reported in up to 55% to 90% of affected patients.[12,13]

The posterior sagittal anorectoplasty (PSARP), first described by Peña and Devries[36] in the 1980s, is still considered the mainstay of therapy for ARM by many pediatric surgeons. The technique, in line with the classification of ARMs, has evolved over the past 3 decades, continuing to reflect the principles of managements that Peña and Devries[36] described.[14,15] Taking the early lessons from Peña and Devries[36] into account, understanding of the functional outcomes, risks, and benefits of various surgical techniques has continued to evolve. Perhaps most importantly, advances in neonatal medicine and laparoscopic technology have made minimally invasive abdominal approaches to ARM a reality.

Laparoscopic-assisted anorectal pull-through (LAARP) was first described and popularized by Georgeson and Inge[17] in 2000, building on prior experience with laparoscopic treatment of Hirschsprung disease.[16,17] Based on a growing body of

Table 1		
Wingspread classification of anorectal malformations (1984)		
	Male	**Female**
High	• Anorectal agenesis • With rectoprostatic urethral fistula • Without fistula • Rectal atresia	• Anorectal agenesis • With rectovaginal fistula • Without fistula • Rectal atresia
Intermediate	• Rectobulbar-urethral fistula • Anal agenesis without fistula	• Rectovestibular fistula • Rectovaginal fistula • Anal agenesis without fistula
Low	• Anocutaneous fistula • Anal stenosis	• Anovestibular fistula • Anocutaneous fistula • Anal stenosis
Rare Malformations		• Cloaca

From Stephens FD, Smith ED, Paoul NW. Anorectal malformations in children: update 1988. March of Dimes Birth Defect Foundation. Original series, vol. 24(4). New York: Alan R Liss; 1988.

literature citing advantages of laparoscopic approaches to other pediatric surgical conditions, the minimally invasive approach to ARM was thought to provide excellent visualization of the rectal fistula and surrounding structures, thus allowing more accurate placement of the pull-through segment at the center of the levator sling.[17–20] More accurate positioning of the anastomosis and the suspected, although unproven, argument that the laparoscopic approach limits damage to the sphincter are frequently cited as benefits of LAARP compared with PSARP.[18] Although the laparoscopic approach offers some advantages, the absence of clearly defined protocols and standards of care has hindered the ability to assess outcomes and draw conclusions between traditional PSARP and LAARP.

INDICATIONS/CONTRAINDICATIONS

Although laparoscopic surgery has been safely performed for well more than 2 decades, its success in all patients, and especially in the neonatal population, is highly dependent on appropriate patient and provider selection. Advanced laparoscopic procedures in the neonatal and pediatric population demand not only acquisition but mastery of surgical techniques only popularized within the past few decades. Several factors delayed the progress of laparoscopic adaptation in pediatric surgery, including the need for specialized equipment, biases against the need for smaller incisions, a gross underestimate of patient discomfort, and a long learning curve.[21,22] The popularity of the LAARP for ARM, described by Georgeson and colleagues,[17] continues to increase in parallel with increased provider familiarity with minimally invasive techniques.

Beyond surgeon comfort, the most frequently cited and indisputable indication for laparoscopy is a case in which the abdomen needs to be entered to repair the malformation.[15,23] Specific considerations and anatomic variants in which this may be the case are described in **Table 2**. Contraindications, aside from anatomic variants not amenable to or necessitating abdominal exposure, are determined by conditions of general physiology. Pending hospital capabilities and surgeon and anesthesiologist comfort levels, patients with severe cardiac disease, bleeding disorders, significant hemodynamic instability, or pulmonary insufficiency may be suboptimal candidates for laparoscopy.[24]

SURGICAL TECHNIQUE/PROCEDURE
Preoperative Planning

As in any surgical procedure, preoperative planning and patient selection are paramount to a successful operation. A full physical examination must be performed at

Table 2
Anatomic considerations for selection of laparoscopic-assisted anorectal pull-through

Amenable to Laparoscopic Approach	Laparoscopy Not Indicated
Male	Rectoperineal fistula
Recto–bladder neck fistula	Rectourethral bulbar fistula
Rectoprostatic fistulas	Rectovestibular fistula
Free-floating rectum	Rectal atresia
Female	Most cloacae
Complex cloacae, common channel >3 cm long	Most ARMs without fistula, if low
Rectovestibular fistula, absent vagina	
Free-floating rectum	

Data from Levitt M, Kim ES. Pediatric imperforate anus surgery treatment & management. 2015. Available at: http://emedicine.medscape.com/article/933524-treatment#d11. Accessed March 19, 2017.

birth for evaluation of ARM and to identify any signs of chromosomal abnormalities or dysmorphic features. Studies directed at the characterization of commonly associated anomalies and specific anatomic features of the ARM are described later.[25] In addition, classification of the presence and type of rectal fistula facilitates meaningful comparison of clinical outcomes and optimal surgical planning.[26]

1. Work-up for associated anomalies.[27]
   a. Cardiac evaluation including echocardiogram.
   b. Spinal radiograph, spinal ultrasonography, or babygram to evaluate for spinal anomalies, including hemivertebrae; MRI may be performed in older patients.
   c. Genitourinary evaluation with renal or abdominal ultrasonography followed by voiding cystourethrogram for abnormalities on screening genitourinary ultrasonography.
   d. Complete physical examination for limb evaluation; plain film radiographs if needed.
2. Work-up for type of ARM, including pressure-augmented fluoroscopic mucous fistulogram with consideration of magnetic resonance (MR) fistulography pending need for spinal MR and associated imaging studies.[28,29]
3. General surgical preoperative care, including relevant laboratory studies and family history.
4. For patients presenting for LAARP following diverting stoma performed in the early perinatal period, consideration should be made for irrigation of distal rectum when possible. In the event that a mucous fistula has been created at the initial operation, mucous fistulogram and irrigations for residual stool may be initiated. Rarely, the authors consider use of a flexible neonatal endoscope in the mucous fistula to evaluate for residual stool and continue irrigation.

Surgical Approach

As noted, surgical approach largely depends on the type of anomaly as determined by the presence of a fistula and rectal stump. The general approach for laparoscopic-assisted anorectal pull-through as may be performed in a male patient with a recto–bladder neck fistula is described here. Depending on overall patient stability and associated anomalies, patients may require a diverting colostomy during the initial neonatal period.[19] In most cases, this protective or diverting colostomy may be created laparoscopically. Although some surgeons prefer a simple loop colostomy, a divided colostomy at the very proximal sigmoid with a distal mucous fistula is the preferred approach and allows for some redundancy in the distal colon, making mobilization of the neorectum down to the perineum easier as well as protecting from any stool spilling over into the urinary tract.[30–32]

1. Patient positioning
   a. The patient should be placed in the supine position toward the foot of the operating room table with appropriate padding of all extremities. Infants can be positioned crosswise on the typical operating room table to allow the surgeon and assistant to more easily stand at the head of the patient and work in line toward the pelvis.
   b. Legs may be placed in low lithotomy or frog-legged position to permit access to the perineum. Alternative positioning, including wrapping the legs in bandages and fixing them above the patient's head to expose the perineum, may be used.
   c. If not already in place, a Foley catheter should be inserted by the surgeon to avoid inadvertent cannulation of fistula. Cystoscopy, when available, may be required to assist in Foley catheter placement.

2. Surgical approach, principles, procedure details[33,34]
   a. Following induction of general anesthesia and possible provision of regional anesthetic, the patient is positioned, prepped, and draped. Although practice patterns may vary, the authors recommend Povidone-iodine or alcohol-based solution from nipples to feet before wrapping legs in sterile bandages and fixing the wraps to the drapes above the patient's head, exposing the perineum when needed.
   b. A muscle stimulator should then be used to clearly delineate the anal and pelvic muscle complexes for precise anatomic placement of the rectal pull-through segment. Before stimulation, the tissue should be moistened with warm saline and the stimulator calibrated to device specifications.[35,36]
   c. Initial access is obtained via a 5-mm port to accommodate a 30° scope via a transumbilical approach.
   d. An additional 5-mm trocar may be placed in the right upper quadrant; 3-mm trocars may be inserted in the left upper and right lower quadrants for instruments.
   e. A stay stitch may be placed through the bladder and/or uterus to suspend the structures anteriorly to the abdominal wall for better pelvic visualization.[37]
   f. Identification of fistula:
      i. The distal rectum is identified near the peritoneal reflection and the peritoneum is divided close to the rectal wall to avoid injury to surrounding structures, including nerves, ureters, and vas deferens. Typically, hook cautery is adequate for this dissection.
      ii. Dissection is continued circumferentially and distally until the bladder neck and fistula are identified. In a bladder neck fistula, the rectum usually joins the urinary tract in a T fashion without a common wall, facilitating easier fistula ligation.
   g. Fistula ligation:
      i. Multiple techniques for ligation exist and selection may depend on institutional and provider preferences.
      ii. An endoloop may be introduced with a Maryland-type clamp passed through the loop.
      iii. The fistula is then divided with scissors and the clamp is used to control the distal fistula at the bladder neck. The endoloop is passed over the clamp and is tightened to close the fistula.
   h. The rectum is further mobilized through division of avascular attachments.
   i. Identification of location of sphincter and preparation of anastomosis.
      i. Perineal approach:
         1. The legs should be elevated and the center of the external sphincter confirmed with the use of an electric Peña nerve stimulator.
         2. A 1-cm vertical incision is made and a fine clamp is used to dissect through the subcutaneous tissue and through the center of the sphincter. A sheath-covered Veress needle can now be passed through this dissection plane, central to the bellies of the right and left pubococcygeus muscle complex and into the pelvic space with laparoscopic visualization guidance. Care must be taken to avoid injury to the urethra or prostate gland. The needle is removed and a 5-mm cannula is passed through the expandable sheath with laparoscopic guidance. The 5-mm cannula is removed and a 10-mm or 12-mm cannula is then passed through the expandable sheath in order to dilate the pathway from the perineum into the pelvis. A grasper is now passed through the trocar and, using laparoscopic assistance, the

divided fistula/distal rectum is grasped and pulled down and through the pathway as the trocar is removed, allowing the rectum to easily reach the perineum. The rectum should not be on tension.
3. Procedure is completed by suturing the open neorectum to the perineal skin central to the external sphincter complex.[36]
   ii. Laparoscopic sphincter identification:
      1. A laparoscopic Peña-type nerve stimulator has been developed and can provide extra information about the exact location, between the bellies of the pubococcygeus complex, of the site for passing the Veress needle from the perineum into the pelvic space.[38]

POSTOPERATIVE CARE

One of the frequently cited limitations of existing review articles on the topic of laparoscopic approaches to ARM is the absence of standardized approaches to postoperative care. There are no published consensus statements on the most appropriate management of these patients, including duration of follow-up and appropriate monitoring adjuncts. Based on review of the literature, the following protocol is proposed to assist in developing a uniform approach that will better position clinicians for future evaluation and comparison of techniques.

Pain Management

When possible, avoidance of narcotics for pain management is recommended in the neonatal and pediatric populations. The laparoscopic approach is thought to be associated with less pain and therefore a shorter length of stay, fewer constipation complications, and decreased need for narcotics.[39] Scheduled acetaminophen and/or administration of intraoperative regional analgesia may assist in perioperative pain management.

Urinary Catheter

Duration of urinary catheter maintenance largely depends on surgeon preference and presence of urinary tract fistula. In most cases, the catheter may be left in for 5 to 14 days, with a longer duration recommended for more complex repairs to prevent leakage of urine through the newly ligated fistula tract and wound breakdown.

Antibiotics

Clear data on routine use of postoperative antibiotics are lacking and their use is determined by provider and institutional policy. Depending on intraoperative complications and contamination, antibiotics such as ampicillin and gentamicin may be administered intravenously for 24 to 72 hours postoperatively.[40]

Feeding

Early initiation of enteric feeds is generally recommended following pediatric surgical procedures. In the case of ARM, the timing depends on resolution of ileus and presence of a diverting or protective ostomy. In the case of a previously functioning ostomy, feeds may be initiated within 24 to 48 hours of the procedure.

Dilatation

Despite the known complication of anal stenosis following perineal repair of ARM, with or without laparoscopic assistance, there is persistent controversy around the practice of anal dilatations. Often cited as a cause of significant stress for children and parents, dilation practices have been linked to impairments in mental health and psychosocial function.[41,42] With these concerns in mind, a survey of European pediatric surgical centers of excellence identified 74% of centers as regularly initiating dilations 2 weeks postoperatively.[15] Limited reports showed similar outcomes between daily dilation by parents and weekly calibration by the surgeon but daily or twice daily dilations are most frequently used.[43]

Timing of Additional Procedures

In general, reversal of a diverting or protective colostomy, in the absence of relevant surgical complications, is performed within 2 to 4 months of the pull-through procedure. Irrigation through functioning and nonfunctioning stoma, if present, is not routinely recommended but may done at the discretion of the surgeon, especially in the setting of loop colostomy. Additional studies, such as contrast enema, are not routinely performed but may help predict success after colostomy closure and need for ongoing dilation.[5]

COMPLICATIONS AND MANAGEMENT

1. Intraoperative complications: type and severity of intraoperative complication and surgeon comfort with minimally invasive procedures determine the need to convert to laparotomy for management of intraoperative complications
   a. Leakage of stool into abdominal cavity: depending on presence of diverting or protective stoma before pull-through procedure, bowel preparation may be performed to reduce the risk of sequelae from leakage. Fecal contamination from the distal colon is reportedly more common in double-barrel colostomy. Leakage may result in need for extended course of antibiotics or procedural intervention if resulting in abscess.[44]
   b. Bleeding: although variable across studies, studies reporting on intraoperative blood loss estimated less blood loss with laparoscopic approaches at an average of 20 ± 5.7 g.[44,45]
   c. Injuries to surrounding structures: injury to ureters, nerves, and vas deferens are minimized by carrying out dissection as close to rectal wall as possible. There are no studies definitely comparing the incidence of ureteral injury between laparoscopic and open surgical approaches for ARM.
   d. Urethral diverticulum: diverticulum may result as a consequence of technical error where a large residual stump of rectourethral fistula is left in place attached to the urethra intraoperatively.
2. Short-term postoperative complications:
   a. Superficial dehiscence of perineal anastomosis (neoanus): although uncommon in LAARP, anastomotic dehiscence causing a perineal wound problem carries high morbidity if the infection corrupts the pelvic floor reconstruction because this may play a significant role in maintenance of long-term fecal continence. Current literature supports a higher rate of wound infection and dehiscence of perineal wounds in patients who underwent PSARP compared with LAARP (11.8% vs 0%)[45] but application of these results to counseling practice is limited by lack of high-quality, randomized controlled, prospective studies.[34,39,46] The presence of a diverting or protective colostomy influences management of wound complications, which ranges from bowel rest and antibiotics to surgical revision or creation of colostomy. The

rate of perineal wound complications is thought to be underreported in the setting of diverting stoma; most perineal wound complications resolve spontaneously.

b. Postoperative urethral diverticulum: as described in multiple articles and addressed in meta-analysis and systematic reviews, urethral diverticulum is thought to be avoided almost entirely when posterior sagittal repair is performed because of the careful dissection required to separate the anterior rectal wall from the posterior urethral wall.[23] Despite advances in the surgical management of ARMs, the reported incidence of urethral diverticula is approximately 17.8%, with increased incidence in male patients.[47] Regardless of type of procedure performed initially, most patients presenting with urethral diverticulum require reoperation and excision, either through a perineal or laparoscopic approach, because of the increased risk of urinary tract infection and calculus formation, and a small incidence of malignant transformation.[48]

c. Urinary retention: transient urinary retention is an uncommon complication reported in less than 10% of patients undergoing laparoscopic-assisted anorectal pull-through.[49] In a review of 34 articles, only 4 cases of urinary retention were reported and the literature presently does not identify a varying rate in this complication between LAARP and traditional PSARP.[50]

d. Other postoperative complications requiring changes in routine medical management by way of extended antibiotics or surgical revision of anastomosis include the rarer, but often very serious, anastomotic leak, pelvic sepsis, and retraction (**Table 3**).[23]

3. Interim complications

a. Colostomy-related complications: a variety of complications may occur in the presence of colostomy, regardless of approach to anorectal pull-through procedure. Most of these complications may be managed in the usual fashion with hope for early reversal following LAARP (**Table 4**).[30]

Table 3 Complications reported in the literature following laparoscopic-assisted anorectal pull-through	
Total complications	74
Rectal prolapse	21
Posterior diverticulum	16
Anal stenosis	11
Peritoneal contamination with fecal material	6
Perineal reoperations	4
Urethral leak	2
Conversion to laparotomy	2
Temporary neurogenic bladder	2
Peritonitis	2
Postoperative dysuria	2
Colitis, bowel perforation, perineal infection, evisceration at trocar site, partial dehiscence, intestinal obstruction caused by adhesions	1 each

From Bischoff A, Levitt M, Pena A. Laparoscopy and its use in the repair of anorectal malformations. J Pediatr Surg 2011;46(8):1609–17.

Table 4
Colostomy-related complications in patients with anorectal malformations

Complication	Characteristics	Management
Colostomy prolapse	Less common in divided stoma	Separate loop colostomy to make divided Early colostomy reversal
Retraction	Less common in loop colostomy Usually associated with nonfunctional stoma, mucous fistula	May require revision of mucous fistula or colostomy
Need for revision	Seen with attempted transverse colostomy and inadvertent malpositioning of descending colostomy in right upper quadrant	Revision often required at time of anorectoplasty

From Bischoff A, Levitt MA, Lawal TA, et al. Colostomy closure: how to avoid complications. Pediatr Surg Int 2010;26(11):1087–92.

b. Anastomotic stricture: reported in the meta-analysis by Bischoff and colleagues,[50] roughly 73.5% of articles reporting complications included postoperative anal stenosis. In this and other reviews, the incidence of anal stenosis is reportedly higher in LAARP than in PSARP but the difference was not statistically significant (risk ratio = 1.32; 95% confidence interval [CI], 0.61–2.86; $P = .48$).[39] The stricture, which usually occurs as fibrosis in the distal rectum secondary to ischemia of distal neorectum or as a skin stricture, occurs with inadequate dilation and is often adequately managed expectantly with anal dilations or postoperatively with dilations under anesthesia. Depending on the degree of stricture and functional implications, repair may involve a formal redo anoplasty or a Heineke-Mikulicz–like stricturoplasty for skin-level stricture.[51]

c. Mucosal prolapse: incidence of mucosal prolapse (17.7% in LAARP and 12.8% in PSARP), although reported in some studies as lower in patients who undergo LAARP compared with PSARP, is poorly evaluated because of significant

Table 5
International classification (Krickenbeck) for postoperative results

1. Voluntary bowel movements	Yes/no
Feeling of urge, capacity to verbalize, hold the bowel movement	
2. Soiling	Yes/no
Grade 1	Occasionally (once or twice per week)
Grade 2	Every day, no social problem
Grade 3	Constant, social problem
3. Constipation	Yes/no
Grade 1	Manageable by changes in diet
Grade 2	Requires laxatives
Grade 3	Resistant to laxatives and diet

From Al-Hozaim O, Al-Maary J, AlQahtani A, et al. Laparoscopic-assisted anorectal pull-through for anorectal malformations: a systematic review and the need for standardization of outcome reporting. J Pediatr Surg 2010;45(7):1500–4.

heterogeneity of low-quality studies and grouping of male and female patients with various defects (risk ratio = 1.23; 95% CI, 0.74–2.02; P = .42).[20] More often than by procedure type, rectal prolapse is reported at a higher rate among patients with associated malformation and poor sacral and pelvic musculature. In some cases, the rate was reportedly reduced by meticulous dissection and rectal fixation with seromuscular sutures between the rectum and presacral fascia.[46,52]

Table 6 Rintala score for evaluation of fecal continence	
Ability to Hold Back Defecation	
Always	3
Problems (<1/wk)	2
Weekly problems	1
No voluntary control	0
Feels/Reports the Urge to Defecate	
Always	3
Most of the time	2
Uncertain	1
Absent	0
Frequency of Defecation	
Every other day to twice a day	2
More often	1
Less often	1
Soiling	
Never	3
Staining <1/wk, no change in underwear required	2
Frequent staining, change of underwear often required	1
Daily soiling, requires protective aids	0
Accidents	
Never	3
Fewer than 1/wk	2
Weekly, often requires protective aids	1
Daily, requires protective aids during day and night	0
Constipation	
No constipation	3
Manageable with diet	2
Manageable with laxatives	1
Manageable with enemas	0
Social Problems	
No social problems	3
Sometimes (foul odors)	2
Problems causing restrictions in social life	1
Severe social and/or psychic problems	0

From Arnoldi R, Macchini F, Gentilino V, et al. Anorectal malformations with good prognosis: variables affecting the functional outcome. J Pediatr Surg 2014;49(8):1232–6.

OUTCOMES

Since first being published by Peña in 1995, and with increasing interest in evidence-based surgery, voluntary bowel movements, soiling, and constipation have been regarded as the main postoperative parameters to evaluate the success of an operation.[53] Although multiple systematic reviews and meta-analyses have attempted to identify differences in outcomes based on type of procedure, the primary differences in outcome are often attributable to the type of malformation, location of fistula, and quality of the sacrum and spine.[33] A standardized approach to assessing postoperative outcomes is recommended in order to draw comparisons between the procedures based on relevant clinical characteristics. A variety of tools, including the international classification (Krickenbeck score; **Table 5**), defecation assessment score, Kelly score, ARM score, fecal continence evaluation questionnaire, and Rintala score are used in the literature, with inconsistent reporting of urologic outcomes and variable duration of follow-up (**Table 6**).[18] The lack of voluntary control of bowel movements at an early age limits the applicability of many of these tools until a later age, at which time follow-up is even less consistent.

It is our recommendation that follow-up be continued indefinitely with appropriate provision of transitional care to adult providers beginning at age 15 years. Ongoing assessment should include a record of the type of malformation; type of procedure performed; need for reoperation or follow-up procedures; and classification of voluntary bowel movements, soiling, and constipation. A cumulative score may then be generated to compare procedures and quality of life for patients with ARM. The routine use of anal pressure measurement and anorectal angulation as determined by barium enema may have academic utility in early attempts to differentiate outcomes of open PSARP and LAARP, although the tests alone do not seem to affect patient outcomes.[49]

SUMMARY

As is often the case in medicine, there is a continuous pattern to the evolution and shaping of paradigms of care within a particular disease process. Not only has the provision of surgical care to neonates evolved technically but advances in the care of children and neonatology have made previously fatal disease processes survivable. Moving beyond survivable, technical advances have enhanced the safety, efficiency, and cosmesis of surgery. Laparoscopy, gaining popularity among pediatric surgeons since the 1990s, has revolutionized many aspects of surgical disease.[54] However, in anorectal malformation, multiple variables remain at play that both limit and enhance the existing data on the use of LAARP procedures for ARM.

PSARP has been the standard technique for the management of ARMs since it was standardized by Peña and Devries[36] in 1982. PSARP, which is often associated with a large gluteal cleft incision and extensive perineal dissection, frequently involves division of muscles with subsequent closure. Occasionally, laparotomy has been used to identify higher fistulas or rectal atresias, which are often associated with poor functional outcomes. Because fistula location is thought to best correlate with functional outcomes, patients who undergo laparotomy for identification of high fistula have also been observed to have worse long-term functional outcomes.

In parallel with evolving laparoscopic techniques, the LAARP gained popularity for improved visualization for high/intermediate ARMs and the potential for more accurate visualization and placement of the neorectum through the pubococcygeus complex and neoanus through the sphincteric complex.[39] Extensive literature reviews have been conducted in an attempt to definitively classify 1 procedure as superior in functional outcomes following repair of ARM. However, most studies reviewed are retrospective, of low to moderate quality, and used inconsistent means of assessing postoperative outcome. The reviews are further limited by the small field of pediatric surgery, such that, in reviewing published articles, it is not possible to determine whether the patients mentioned in various publications by the same investigators are represented more than once.[50]

Despite obvious limitations, it is the recommendation of the authors after thorough literature review that the primary indication for laparoscopy is in place of laparotomy and when a high to intermediate ARM defect is suspected.[18] Particularly in the case of recto–bladder neck and rectoprostatic fistula, the technical advantages of LAARP are well described. However, the results and use depend greatly on surgeon level of expertise. There is no significant difference in rates of mucosal prolapse or defecation scores for LAARP compared with perineal repair based on heterogeneous studies without standardization of postoperative guidelines.[20]

Although the potential advantages of LAARP are clear, a possible explanation for the difficulty in showing improved outcomes lies in the patient selection. As noted, LAARP is most strongly indicated in cases of high or intermediate defects. However, more severe defects are most often associated with spinal anomalies and poor functional outcomes, regardless of surgical technique. In one study addressing the utility of anorectal manometry to assess functional outcomes, findings correlated most closely with type of ARM rather than repair.[55,56] Secondary outcomes, such as mean operative time, hospital length of stay, recurrent fistula, and general wound complications, are reportedly superior in LAARP compared with PSARP.[45]

In contrast, for low defects in which rectourethral bulbar fistula is suspected or visualized on preoperative imaging, LAARP is possible but careful attention must be paid to avoid a urethral diverticulum resulting from suboptimal fistula resection. This type of ARM may be more readily approached through a posterior sagittal incision in which the long wall between the rectum and urethra is separated perineally rather than from an abdominal approach with laparoscopy or laparotomy.[48,57]

Another shift that may, in part, be attributable to the increased use of minimally invasive surgery in the management of ARM is the timing of intervention. Primary repair has long been reserved for patients with a low malformation or perineal fistula amenable to PSARP with minimal perineal dissection. Alternatively, early neonatal colostomy, via an open or laparoscopic procedure, is used for initial management of high malformation. Some studies show improved functional outcomes by Rintala score and anorectal manometry for patients who undergo immediate repair.[56] However, as noted, the defects present in these patients, and therefore other clinical characteristics, are innately different and influence functional outcomes, thereby confounding the ability to attribute results to timing of operation alone.[58,59]

The absence of standardized recommendations for follow-up is the greatest limiting factor in definitively comparing LAARP and PSARP. From fecal continence evaluation questionnaires to detailed assessments of perineal erosion, frequency of defecation, staining/soiling, and need for medication, a variety of tools exist.[57] It is our recommendation that, in addition to an individualized approach to patient selection for laparoscopy, standardized guidelines are needed to evaluate functional outcomes using clinical, manometric, and radiological studies.[19]

Best Practices

What is the current practice?

1. Neonates diagnosed with ARM, including imperforate anus, require thorough investigation for concurrent anomalies as well as diagnostic studies to characterize ARM.

2. There are no randomized controlled trials addressing the type of repair, including traditional PSARP versus LAARP, for ARM.

3. Meta-analyses and systematic reviews identify some advantages to LAARP with regard to length of stay, decreased incidence of mucosal prolapse, and suspected improved functional outcomes. These studies are limited by heterogeneity of inclusion criteria and specific ARM.

4. Close follow-up and standardized functional assessments are mandatory to appropriately differentiate between outcomes attributable to surgical intervention and outcomes attributable to defect anatomy.

What changes in current practice are likely to improve outcomes?

1. Active clinical research, including a randomized controlled trial, at a center where providers are proficient in both minimally invasive and open approaches to ARM are needed to develop evidence-based practice recommendations that specifically seek to optimize functional outcomes.

2. A standardized approach to follow-up and assessment of functional outcomes should include bowel habit scores and diagnostic imaging studies to further clarify the efficacy of the various surgical approaches.

3. A clinical algorithm is needed to standardize care; however, given the fairly recent application of LAARP to ARM, surgeon comfort and familiarity with the techniques involved must be addressed.

Strength of evidence

B: recommendations based on inconsistent or limited-quality patient-oriented evidence

Summary statement

The management of ARM has many unanswered questions despite recent advances in functional analysis and minimally invasive surgical techniques. Many advantages have been observed anecdotally and are hypothesized with the LAARP but, given the variability in outcomes by type of ARM, and not necessarily by surgical approach, further research is needed to understand how the intervention affects short-term and long-term postoperative function.

REFERENCES

1. Aegineta P, Adams F. On the imperforate anus. The seven books (book 6). London: Sydenham Society; 1844.

2. Lau PE, Cruz S, Cassady CI, et al. Prenatal diagnosis and outcome of fetal gastrointestinal obstruction. J Pediatr Surg 2017;52(5):722–5.

3. Moore SW, Alexander A, Sidler D, et al. The spectrum of anorectal malformations in Africa. Pediatr Surg Int 2008;24(6):677–83.

4. Alves JC, Sidler D, Lotz JW, et al. Comparison of MR and fluoroscopic mucous fistulography in the pre-operative evaluation of infants with anorectal malformation: a pilot study. Pediatr Radiol 2013;43(8):958–63.

5. Levitt MA, Peña A. Anorectal malformations. Orphanet J Rare Dis 2007;2:33.

6. Torres R, Levitt MA, Tovilla JM, et al. Anorectal malformations and Down's syndrome. J Pediatr Surg 1998;33(2):194–7.

7. Steinbok P, Garton HJ, Gupta N. Occult tethered cord syndrome: a survey of practice patterns. J Neurosurg 2006;104(5 Suppl):309–13.

8. Levitt MA, Patel M, Rodriguez G, et al. The tethered spinal cord in patients with anorectal malformations. J Pediatr Surg 1997;32(3):462–8.

9. Solomon BD, Baker LA, Bear KA, et al. An approach to the identification of anomalies and etiologies in neonates with identified or suspected VACTERL (vertebral defects, anal atresia, tracheo-esophageal fistula with esophageal atresia, cardiac anomalies, renal anomalies, and limb anomalies) association. J Pediatr 2014; 164(3):451–7.e1.

10. Solomon BD. VACTERL/VATER association. Orphanet J Rare Dis 2011;6:56.

11. Stoll C, Alembik Y, Dott B, et al. Associated malformations in patients with anorectal anomalies. Eur J Med Genet 2007;50(4):281–90.

12. Levitt MA, Peña A. Cloacal malformations: lessons learned from 490 cases. Semin Pediatr Surg 2010;19(2):128–38.

13. Rich MA, Brock WA, Pena A. Spectrum of genitourinary malformations in patients with imperforate anus. Pediatr Surg Int 1988;3:110–3.

14. Oral A, Caner I, Yigiter M, et al. Clinical characteristics of neonates with VACTERL association. Pediatr Int 2012;54(3):361–4.

15. Morandi A, Ure B, Leva E, et al. Survey on the management of anorectal malformations (ARM) in European pediatric surgical centers of excellence. Pediatr Surg Int 2015;31(6):543–50.

16. Willital G. Endosurgical intrapuborectal reconstruction of high anorectal anomalies. Pediatr Endosurg Innov Tech 1998;2(1):5–11. Available at: http://online.liebertpub.com/doi/abs/10.1089/pei.1998.2.5. Accessed October 5, 2017.

17. Georgeson KE, Inge TH, Albanese CT. Laparoscopically assisted anorectal pull-through for high imperforate anus–a new technique. J Pediatr Surg 2000;35(6): 927–30 [discussion: 930–1].

18. Al-Hozaim O, Al-Maary J, AlQahtani A, et al. Laparoscopic-assisted anorectal pull-through for anorectal malformations: a systematic review and the need for standardization of outcome reporting. J Pediatr Surg 2010;45(7):1500–4.

19. Ruggeri G, Destro F, Randi B, et al. Laparoscopic-assisted anorectal pull-through for high imperforate anus: 14 years experience in a single center. J Laparoendosc Adv Surg Tech A 2016;26(5):404–8.

20. Shawyer A, Livingston M, Cook D, et al. Laparoscopic versus open repair of recto-bladderneck and recto-prostatic anorectal malformations: a systematic review and meta-analysis. Pediatr Surg Int 2017;31:17–30.

21. Georgeson K, Owings E. Advances in minimally invasive surgery in children. Am J Surg 2000;180(5):362–4.

22. Esposito C, Escolino M, Draghici I, et al. Training models in pediatric minimally invasive surgery: rabbit model versus porcine model: a comparative study. J Laparoendosc Adv Surg Tech A 2016;26(1):79–84.

23. Bischoff A, Levitt M, Pena A. Laparoscopy and its use in the repair of anorectal malformations. J Pediatr Surg 2011;46(8):1609–17.

24. Truchon R. Anaesthetic considerations for laparoscopic surgery in neonates and infants: a practical review. Best Pract Res Clin Anaesthesiol 2004;18(2):343–55.

25. Nah S, Ong C, Lakshmi N, et al. Anomalies associated with anorectal malformations according to the Krickenbeck anatomic classification. J Pediatr Surg 2012; 47(12):2273–8.

26. Yang J, Zhang W, Feng J, et al. Comparison of clinical outcomes and anorectal manometry in patients with congenital anorectal malformations treated with

posterior sagittal anorectoplasty and laparoscopically assisted anorectal pull through. J Pediatr Surg 2009;44(12):2380–3.

27. Lane V, Ambeba E, Chisolm D, et al. Low vertebral ano-rectal cardiac tracheo-esophageal renal limb screening rates in children with anorectal malformations. J Surg Res 2016;203(2):398–406.

28. Gross GW, Wolfson PJ, Pena A. Augmented-pressure colostogram in imperforate anus with fistula. Pediatr Radiol 1991;21(8):560–2.

29. Alamo L, Meyrat BJ, Meuwly JY, et al. Anorectal malformations: finding the pathway out of the labyrinth. Radiographics 2013;33(2):491–512.

30. Almosallam OI, Aseeri A, Shanafey SA. Outcome of loop versus divided colostomy in the management of anorectal malformations. Ann Saudi Med 2016;36(5):352–5.

31. Oda O, Davies D, Colapinto K, et al. Loop versus divided colostomy for the management of anorectal malformations. J Pediatr Surg 2014;49(1):87–90 [discussion: 90].

32. Youssef F, Arbash G, Puligandla PS, et al. Loop versus divided colostomy for the management of anorectal malformations: a systematic review and meta-analysis. J Pediatr Surg 2017;52(5):783–90.

33. Bischoff A, Pena A, Levitt M. Laparoscopic-assisted PSARP — the advantages of combining both techniques for the treatment of anorectal malformations with recto-bladderneck or high prostatic fistulas. J Pediatr Surg 2013;48(2):367–71.

34. Bailez MM, Cuenca ES, Di Benedetto V, et al. Laparoscopic treatment of rectovaginal fistulas. Feasibility, technical details, and functional results of a rare anorectal malformation. J Pediatr Surg 2010;45(9):1837–42.

35. Short S, Kimble K, Zhai S, et al. A low-cost improvised nerve stimulator is equivalent to high-cost muscle stimulator for anorectal malformation surgery. Eur J Pediatr Surg 2012;23:025–8.

36. Peña A, Devries PA. Posterior sagittal anorectoplasty: important technical considerations and new applications. J Pediatr Surg 1982;17(6):796–811.

37. Liem NT, Quynh TA. Combined laparoscopic and modified posterior sagittal approach saving the external sphincter for rectourethral fistula: an easier and more physiologic approach. J Pediatr Surg 2013;48(6):1450–3.

38. Lima M, Tursini S, Ruggeri G, et al. Laparoscopically assisted anorectal pull-through for high imperforate anus: three years' experience. J Laparoendosc Adv Surg Tech A 2006;16(1):63–6.

39. Han Y, Xia Z, Guo S, et al. Laparoscopically assisted anorectal pull-through versus posterior sagittal anorectoplasty for high and intermediate anorectal malformations: a systematic review and meta-analysis. PLoS One 2017;12(1):e0170421.

40. Colorectal Center at Cincinnati Children's. Postoperation care after pull-through/PSARP surgery for anorectal malformations/imperforate anus. Available at: https://www.cincinnatichildrens.org/-/media/cincinnati%20childrens/home/service/c/colorectal/treatments/psarp/pull-through-article-1-postop-care-pdf.pdf?la=en. Accessed March 19, 2017.

41. Diseth TH, Egeland T, Emblem R. Effects of anal invasive treatment and incontinence on mental health and psychosocial functioning of adolescents with Hirschsprung's disease and low anorectal anomalies. J Pediatr Surg 1998;33(3):468–75.

42. Diseth TH. Dissociation following traumatic medical treatment procedures in childhood: a longitudinal follow-up. Dev Psychopathol 2006;18(1):233–51.

43. Temple SJ, Shawyer A, Langer JC. Is daily dilatation by parents necessary after surgery for Hirschsprung disease and anorectal malformations? J Pediatr Surg 2012;47(1):209–12.

44. Minaev S, Kirgizoz I, Gladkyy A, et al. Outcome of laparoscopic treatment of anorectal malformations in children. World J Surg 2017;41(2):625–9.
45. Ming A, Li L, Diao M, et al. Long term outcomes of laparoscopic-assisted anorectoplasty: a comparison study with posterior sagittal anorectoplasty. J Pediatr Surg 2014;49(4):560–3.
46. Yazaki Y, Koga H, Ochi T, et al. Surgical management of recto-prostatic and recto-bulbar anorectal malformations. Pediatr Surg Int 2016;32:939–44.
47. Hong AR, Acuña MF, Peña A, et al. Urologic injuries associated with repair of anorectal malformations in male patients. J Pediatr Surg 2002;37(3):339–44.
48. Alam S, Lawal TA, Peña A, et al. Acquired posterior urethral diverticulum following surgery for anorectal malformations. J Pediatr Surg 2011;46(6):1231–5.
49. Kimura O, Iwai N, Sasaki Y, et al. Laparoscopic versus open abdominoperineal rectoplasty for infants with high-type anorectal malformation. J Pediatr Surg 2010;45(12):2390–3.
50. Bischoff A, Martinez-Leo B, Pena A. Laparoscopic approach in the management of anorectal malformations. Pediatr Surg Int 2015;31(5):431–7.
51. Lawal TA, Reck CA, Wood RJ, et al. Use of a Heineke-Mikulicz like stricturoplasty for intractable skin level anal strictures following anoplasty in children with anorectal malformations. J Pediatr Surg 2016;51(10):1743–5.
52. Leung J, Chung P, Tam P, et al. Application of anchoring stitch prevents rectal prolapse in laparoscopic assisted anorectal pullthrough. J Pediatr Surg 2016;51(12):2113–6.
53. Pena A. Anorectal malformations. Semin Pediatr Surg 1995;4:35–47.
54. McBride CA, Holland AJ. Theatre of paediatric surgery. J Paediatr Child Health 2015;51(1):98–102.
55. Kyrklund K, Pakarinen M, Rintala R. Manometric findings in relation to functional outcomes in different types of anorectal malformations. J Pediatr Surg 2017;52(4):563–8.
56. Rintala RJ, Lindahl H. Is normal bowel function possible after repair of intermediate and high anorectal malformations? J Pediatr Surg 1995;30(3):491–4.
57. Koga H, Ochi T, Okawada M, et al. Comparison of outcomes between laparoscopy-assisted and posterior sagittal anorectoplasties for male imperforate anus with recto-bulbar fistula. J Pediatr Surg 2014;49(12):1815–7.
58. Arnoldi R, Macchini F, Gentilino V, et al. Anorectal malformations with good prognosis: variables affecting the functional outcome. J Pediatr Surg 2014;49(8):1232–6.
59. Holschneider A, Hutson J, Peña A, et al. Preliminary report on the International Conference for the Development of Standards for the Treatment of Anorectal Malformations. J Pediatr Surg 2005;40(10):1521–6.

Minimally Invasive Management for Vesicoureteral Reflux in Infants and Young Children

CrossMark

Chung-Kwong Yeung, MD, PhD, FRCS, FRACS[a],*,
Sujit K. Chowdhary, MCh, FRCS[b], Biji Sreedhar, PhD[c]

KEYWORDS

- Vesicoureteric reflux • Antenatal hydronephrosis • Voiding cystourethrography
- Management • Infants • Children • Minimally invasive procedures
- Urinary tract infection

KEY POINTS

- The primary goal in the management of infants with Vesicoureteric reflux (VUR) is to prevent further urinary tract infection and its associated renal damage.
- Minimally invasive ureteral reimplantation is a very attractive and useful tool in the armamentarium for the management of pediatric VUR.
- Subureteric dextranomer injection, laparoscopic extravesical and intravesical ureteric reimplantation with or without robotic assistance are established minimally invasive surgical approaches.

INTRODUCTION

Vesicoureteric reflux (VUR) is a common pediatric problem affecting 1% to 3% of all infants and children. Urinary tract infection (UTI) is the most common presenting symptom of VUR. With the advent of fetal ultrasonogram (USG), antenatal diagnosis of hydronephrosis has increased many-fold and up to 30% of the children with antenatal hydronephrosis have been found to have VUR. Unfortunately, the degree of hydronephrosis on USG does not correlate with the presence or severity of reflux and a normal postnatal USG does not exclude VUR.[1,2] The revised UTI guidelines from the American Academy of Pediatrics state that febrile infants with UTI should undergo USG, although voiding cystourethrography (VCUG) is not recommended

[a] Department of Surgery, University of Hong Kong, 2/F, Professorial Block, Queen Mary Hospital, 102 Pokfulam Road, Hong Kong SAR, China; [b] Pediatric Urology and Pediatric Surgery, Apollo Institute of Pediatric Sciences, Sarita Vihar, Delhi Mathura Road, New Delhi 110076, India; [c] School of Biomedical Sciences, The Chinese University of Hong Kong, Shatin, New Territories, Hong Kong
* Corresponding author.
E-mail address: yeungchungkwong@gmail.com

Clin Perinatol 44 (2017) 835–849
http://dx.doi.org/10.1016/j.clp.2017.08.008
0095-5108/17/© 2017 Elsevier Inc. All rights reserved.

routinely after the first febrile UTI.[3] Because VCUG is a relatively invasive test with higher radiation exposure, the National Institute for Health and Care Excellence guidelines recommended full evaluation with VCUG and dimercaptosuccinic acid (DMSA) scan only in the presence of atypical or recurrent UTI in infants less than 6 months of age.[4] The DMSA scan first, top-down approach pioneered by Hansson and associates[5] helps a lot of children to avoid VCUG and has been regarded by many to be the recommended approach. Although the American Academy of Pediatrics and the National Institute for Health and Care Excellence guidelines recommend further evaluation only for atypical UTI, in places where follow-up compliance is poor, it is probably advisable to evaluate them after a first episode of febrile UTI. In addition, if the desired therapeutic effect cannot be achieved with an initial course of antibiotic treatment, an early VCUG can also be done without a mandatory waiting period.

The primary goal in the management of an infant with VUR is to prevent further UTI and its associated acquired renal damage, and to minimize the morbidity of treatment and follow-up. Just as the spectrum of the disease is very wide, so are the management options, which vary from a conservative observational approach to definitive antireflux surgical treatment. Over the past decades, better understanding of the pathophysiology of the VUR and reflux nephropathy has significantly limited the indication for surgical intervention. Traditionally, management options consist of either conservative treatment with long-term antibiotic prophylaxis or open bladder antireflux surgery. The traditional open bladder surgery is an invasive and traumatic procedure. Although it boasts the advantage of a high cure rate of more than 90%, the intravesical reimplantation technique involves splitting open the abdominal wall and a forced retraction of the bladder. Moreover, urinary diversion with urethral and/or suprapubic catheterization is usually required in the postoperative period, and this measure is associated with a high incidence of significant bladder spasms, leading to severe pain and a prolonged duration of hospital stay.

The introduction of minimally invasive surgical (MIS) techniques has dramatically modified the management strategy for VUR. Various MIS techniques and procedures have been described for the correction of VUR. These include endoscopic subureteral injection of bulking agents referred to as subureteral Teflon injection (STING), and various laparoscopic techniques of ureteral reimplantation, including intravesical, extravesical, and combined procedures. With the advent of robotics technology, different techniques of robotic assisted laparoscopic ureteral reimplantation have also been described. Compared with traditional open surgery, the laparoscopic or MIS approach offers potential superiority and advantages including reduced postoperative pain, shorter duration of hospital stay, quicker return to normal activities, and better cosmesis. Several studies comparing the outcomes of open as well as laparoscopic ureteral reimplantation for VUR had confirmed the safety and feasibility of the latter, and have suggested that the MIS approach should be the preferred technique. Nevertheless, performance of ureteral reimplantation using the MIS approach requires a high degree of surgical precision and advanced laparoscopic technical skills. Great intraoperative care with fine dissection is required during mobilization of the ureters, and caution needs to be taken to prevent damage to the ureteral vascularity, which may lead to ureteric necrosis and strictures in the postoperative period. The advent of robotic assistance has ameliorated some of these technical challenges and has further enhanced the adoption of the minimally invasive approach for definitive treatment for complicated VUR in infants and young children.

In this article, we review the current status of MIS treatment for VUR, and compare the results and efficacies of different laparoscopic ureteral reimplantation techniques (intravesical vs extravesical) with or without robotic assistance.

SURGICAL MANAGEMENT OF VESICOURETERIC REFLUX

The International Reflux Society grading system is widely used as a guide in diagnosis and grading of VUR. Grade 1 to 2 reflux is generally managed conservatively even without antibiotic prophylaxis. The American Urology Association guidelines[6] recommended continuous antibiotic prophylaxis for grades 3 to 5 VUR as initial management. A curative surgical intervention (ureteral reimplantation or STING) may be considered in higher VUR grades and in the presence of scarring. The current indications for surgical intervention in an infant or young child with VUR are as follows: breakthrough UTIs, worsening of renal scars, bilateral grades 4 to 5 VUR, and persistent reflux beyond 4 years of age. For those with unilateral VUR on VCUG, intervention for the contralateral side is preferable when there is opposite kidney scarring on DMSA scan, dilated opposite side ureteric orifice on cystoscopy, or evidence of bilateral reflex on a previous VCUG.

With the introduction of a new MIS concept for reflux treatment the number of STING procedures for reflux has increased, and open surgery rates have remained stable, as reported in a US database study in 2006.[7] However, a later study concluded that the endoscopic management is on the decline, and open surgery rates for VUR were the same.[8] Endoscopic injection (STING) may be useful in grade 3 VUR, with a success rate for reflux resolution of greater than 70%. In those with grades 4 and 5 VUR, the success rate of STING procedure is lower and ureteral reimplantation may be preferred. Until recently, open ureteral reimplantation has remained the benchmark in definitive surgical treatment of VUR, although an MIS approach with the laparoscopic and robotic assisted techniques have also reported comparable success rates. Management of a small infant with VUR and recurrent breakthrough UTI can be more challenging. In general, ureteral reimplantation is avoided in those less than 6 months of age because the bladder may not be large enough for an adequate submucous tunnel. Preferred temporizing options in this setting include continuous medical management, circumcision (in male infants), a STING procedure to cure or downgrade VUR, or a ureterostomy/vesicostomy as a last resort. Follow-up evaluation after endoscopic injection or ureteral reimplantation should include an USG plus a study to look for obstruction or persistent reflux, 3 to 6 months after the procedure. A nuclear renogram with an indirect cystogram (voiding phase to look for VUR) works as an ideal single study in this regard. In places where this is not available, an USG and VCUG can be performed to assess success after the intervention.

ENDOSCOPIC INJECTION OF BULKING AGENT

The endoscopic treatment with subureteral injection of bulking agents under cystoscopic guidance is an appealing option because it is minimally invasive, can be performed on an outpatient basis, has low complication rate, and has a relatively short learning curve. The principle is to create a solid support behind the intravesical ureter at the level of the ureteral orifice, and to elongate the intramural ureter. The STING procedure was originally described by Puri and O'Donnell in 1984[9] and has been used as the representative technique with little modifications over the years. Under cystoscopic guidance, a 3.7-Fr needle is inserted into the bladder mucosa 2 to 3 mm below the ureteric orifice at the 6-o'clock position. The needle is then advanced in the submucosal plane for 4 to 5 mm and a mound is raised by injecting the bulking agent. Various bulking agents have been used but over the last decade, dextranomer/hyaluronic acid (Deflux) has been the most widely used agent for injection therapy. Since its first description, this technique has gained great popularity because it was minimally invasive, easy to learn, and had high patient satisfaction.

However, none of the subsequently reported studies approached the cure rate of open surgery. A metaanalysis conducted by Elder and colleagues[10,11] showed success rates of 57% to 77% for a single injection. The overall reflux resolution rate was 72%. Late recurrence of VUR, ureteral obstruction, and poor efficacy in higher grade reflux have been reported after the endoscopic injection treatment. Despite these limitations, this therapeutic modality has an important role as a first-line surgical treatment for VUR in light of recent studies reporting low effectiveness of antibiotic prophylaxis and concerns about antibiotic-resistant strains, especially for milder grades and during early infancy.

LAPAROSCOPIC EXTRAVESICAL URETERIC REIMPLANTATION

The Lich-Gregoir procedure with extravesical detrusorraphy is the most common technique of extravesical ureteric reimplantation.[12] This procedure involves ureteral hiatal recession by extramucosal tunneling of the ureter into the detrusor. Among all ureteral reimplantation procedures described for correction of VUR, the Lich-Gregoir technique lends itself as technically most easy under the laparoscopic approach. The results of open surgery for VUR by Lich-Gregoir technique have been reported to vary from 95% to 100% in various reports.[12] After attaining such excellent results with open surgery, the focus of management has naturally shifted toward approaches that might minimize surgical morbidity. The laparoscopic approach was the natural evolution toward the minimally invasive treatment concept as a corollary to these efforts.

Technique of Laparoscopic Lich-Gregoir Procedure

The patient is usually admitted the evening before surgery. Gut preparation is done with a dose of mild laxative and enema in the morning on the day of surgery. After general anesthesia and endotracheal intubation, the patient is placed in a low lithotomy position. A cystoscopy is done and urethral catheter placed. The video monitor is positioned at the foot end of the patient, the surgeon stands on the left side of the patient. For infants and younger children, the surgeon can stand at the head end of the table. The camera port is placed at the umbilicus by open technique and pneumoperitoneum with CO_2 is created up to 10 mm Hg pressure. Two working ports are then placed under laparoscopic vision in the right and the left iliac fossa. A stay suture is placed percutaneously and passed through the bladder wall for traction. The bladder is half-filled with saline to aid in dissection. The ureter is dissected from the lateral pelvic fascia for a tension-free reimplantation. The neurovascular bundle of the lower ureter and the vas are protected during this step. The detrusor is then split using an electrocautery hook and blunt dissection, with care taken not to perforate the bladder mucosa. Controlled saline filling and distension of the bladder helps in this part of the dissection, and the mucosa starts to pout through the divided detrusor. A 3- to 4-cm long tunnel is thus created by dividing the detrusor muscle. Thickened bladders owing to recurrent UTI need special handling because they have a higher chance of inadvertent opening of the bladder mucosa. Once an adequate length of tunnel is created, the ureter is placed in the trough and the tension on the ureter is assessed. This is of particular importance in lower grades of VUR, where the ureter is not greatly tortuous and inadequate mobilization of lower ureter can put undue tension over the ureter, which may cause kinking and subsequent obstruction of the ureter at the new hiatus. The ureter is then held in a vascular sling and gentle traction is given by the assistant to maintain the position of ureter in the detrusor trough. This external traction minimizes the handling of the ureter. The split detrusor is now reapproximated over the ureter with interrupted 3-0 or 4-0 polydioxanone sutures. At the completion of the procedure, the bladder is filled with contrast and resolution of VUR confirmed under an image intensifier. The urethral catheter is left in place for 24 hours. No drains are placed.

Using the laparoscopic extravesical (Lich-Gregoir) technique for ureteral reimplantation, various investigators have reported good results, with reflux resolution rates ranging from 92% to 100% (**Table 1**).

LAPAROSCOPIC INTRAVESICAL REIMPLANTATION

The open intravesical approach for ureteral reimplantation has been considered as the gold standard for surgical treatment of VUR. However, the laparoscopic version for intravesical ureteral reimplantation under CO_2 bladder insufflation, or pneumovesicum, was technically more demanding and had a rather steep learning curve. As a result, the extravesical ureteral reimplantation technique has become the preferred laparoscopic approach for the treatment of VUR. The intravesical approach had been described by a small number of authors from selected centers and was effective in their hands, but had never gained wide popularity because of technical reasons.

Technique of Intravesical Ureteral Reimplantation

The preoperative workup and preparation are the same, irrespective of the surgical approach. After general anesthesia and endotracheal intubation, the patient is placed in a low lithotomy position, which allows the procedure to start with cystoscopy. The camera is placed toward the foot end and the surgeon stands at the head end for small children and on left side for older children. The bladder is filled with saline and a stay suture is passed percutaneously at the bladder dome over the site of intended camera port placement under cystoscopic guidance. The first port (for the camera) is placed under cystoscopic vision with saline distension of the bladder. The bladder is then drained and a urethral catheter is inserted and carbon dioxide bladder insufflation (pneumovesicum) is started at pressure of 10 to 12 mm Hg. Endoscopic vision of the inside of the bladder is now established under CO_2 pneumovesicum. Two 3- to

	No. of Patients	No. of Ureters	Mean Age (y)	Mean Follow-up (mo)	Reflux Resolution (%)	Reported Complications
Study						
Marotte & Smith,[12] 2001	44	67	4.7	9.1	92.3	UTI (1 patient), Transient urinary retention (1 patient)
Janetschek et al,[24] 1995	6	9	6–10 (range)	—	100	UTI (1 patient)
Lopez & Varlet,[26] 2010	30	43	4.3	11	100 (ureters)	Postoperative voiding dysfunction (1 patient)
Riquelme et al,[27] 2013	81	95	—	12	96	Nil

Table 1
Studies on laparoscopic extravesical (Lich-Gregoir) ureteral reimplantation for pediatric VUR

Abbreviations: UTI, urinary tract infection; VUR, vesicoureteric reflux.

5-mm working ports are then placed under endoscopic at the lateral walls of the bladder. A percutaneously passed stay suture is used to secure each the port to the bladder as well as the abdominal wall, and will be used to close the port site upon completion of the surgical procedure.

The ureteric orifices are cannulated with a 4- or 6-Fr ureteric catheter to help in ureteral mobilization and dissection. In general, 3-mm laparoscopic instruments are used. The ureter is mobilized using a combination of the diathermy hook and laparoscopic scissors, with sharp and blunt dissection. The ureter is mobilized for a length of 2 to 3 cm into the extravesical space, with special caution being taken to avoid damage of the vascularity of the ureter. The ureteral hiatus is then closed using interrupted 4-0 or 5-0 polydioxanone sutures. Submucosal tunneling is then performed as in the open Cohen's procedure, using a combination of dissection with scissors and diathermy hook cautery. The site of ureteroneocystostomy is chosen usually just lateral and above the contralateral ureteric orifice. The mobilized ureter is pulled through the submucosal tunnel and ureteroneocystostomy performed with interrupted 5-0 or 6-0 polydioxanone sutures. A ureteral stent is usually placed for a period of 4 to 6 weeks. After removal of the ports, the stay sutures at the port entry sites are tied to avoid urine extravasation, and absorbable skin sutures placed. Urethral drainage with catheter is required for 24 to 48 hours.

Using the intravesical technique for cross-trigonal ureteral reimplantation under CO_2 pneumovesicum, various workers have also reported good results, with reflux resolution rates ranging from 93% to 96% (**Table 2**).

ROBOTIC URETERIC REIMPLANTATION

Robotic assistance has helped to overcome some technical limitations of laparoscopic surgery and has gradually gained wider application in the pediatric population. With its 3-dimensional endoscopic vision, elimination of paradoxic movements, and enhanced dexterity with the "endo-wrist" technology, robotic ureteral reimplantation has now become the standard antireflux surgical technique in many centers. The robotic ureteral reimplantation procedure is essentially the same as the laparoscopic procedure. The difference is in that the surgeon now operates through a computer interface that controls the robotic end-effectors inside the patient's body. The

Table 2
Studies on endoscopic cross-trigonal ureteral reimplantation for pediatric VUR

Study	No. of Patients	No. of Ureters	Mean Age (y)	Mean Follow-up (mo)	Reflux Resolution (%)	Reported Complications
Yeung et al,[13] 2005	16	23	4.1	3	96 (ureters)	Nil
Valla et al,[15] 2007	80	131	4.3	31	95 (ureters)	UTI (3 patients)
Kutikov et al,[16] 2006	32	—	—	—	93	Postoperative urinary leak (4 patients), ureteral stricture at the neoureterovesical anastomosis in 2

Abbreviations: UTI, urinary tract infection; VUR, vesicoureteric reflux.

computer sensors of the robotic machine can reliably and delicately translate the movements of the surgeon's fingers and wrists into movements of the slave laparoscopic instruments. The latter are equipped with endo-wrist technology that can execute refined articulated movements with 7° of freedom inside the patient's body cavity. Enhanced visualization and improved dexterity together allow more delicate tissue handling, accurate dissection, and suturing.

The surgical techniques, patient position, and port placement are almost identical in both laparoscopic and robotic ureteral reimplantation, although the robotic approach has in general a longer operating time than the laparoscopic approach. There are a few minor modifications required for the robotic technique. The patient needs extra protective padding over exposed areas to prevent inadvertent injury from the rapidly moving robotic arms. An extra port is placed in the suprapubic area for the assistant to feed the sutures, suctioning, and apply external traction if needed.

The intravesical robotic approach is limited by the small size of pediatric bladder as well as difficulty in maintaining carbon dioxide pneumovesicum. These conditions together cause very significant restriction of manipulation and articulation of the robotic instruments inside the small bladder cavity. These limitations will remain until further miniaturization of the robotic instruments is available. Despite the disadvantages, there are several authors who have reported their experience with intravesical ureteral reimplantation by the robotic approach, although the majority of authors have adopted the extravesical approach for ureteral reimplantation, because the latter has much less limitation by the small size of the pediatric patient. For an intravesical approach, it is recommended that the child should be at least 4 years old with a bladder capacity of more than 200 mL.

With the availability of robotic assistance, various studies have reported successful performance of laparoscopic extravesical (Lich-Gregoir) ureteral reimplantation, although the results were more variable, with reflux resolution rates ranging from 77% to 99% (**Table 3**). There were fewer reports on robotic-assisted intravesical ureteral reimplantation under CO_2 pneumovesicum.

DISCUSSION

Over the past few decades, the management approach to infants and young children with complicated VUR has undergone paradigm shift from an initially primary surgery approach to a mainly conservative approach with continuous antibiotic prophylaxis. With the advent of MIS treatment in the late 1980s, there has been a surge of interest and increasing popularity, first with the endoscopic subureteral injection technique, then to the laparoscopic or robotic-assisted ureteral reimplantation. The pendulum then has most recently swung to a more active surveillance approach without even antibiotic prophylaxis in asymptomatic patients. The spectrum of surgical options now available include the classical open approach using Cohen or Politano-Leadbetter ureteral reimplantation, endoscopic injection of bulking agents, and laparoscopic ureteral reimplantation either using an extravesical approach with the Lich-Gregoir technique, or with an intravesical approach under CO_2 pneumovesicum as described by Yeung and colleagues,[13] with or without robotic assistance.

Cross-trigonal ureteral reimplantation is a time-tested and a most commonly performed procedure for the correction of VUR. A "vesicoscopic" technique for ureteral reimplantation is analogous to standard open cross-trigonal repair in principle, except that it is performed under endoscopic vision using the MIS technique with CO_2 insufflation of the bladder. The pneumovesicoscopic technique uses the fact that the bladder is a naturally distensible cavity and would allow insufflation with gas. The

Table 3
Studies on pediatric extravesical robot-assisted laparoscopic ureteral reimplantation

Study	No. of Patients	No. of Ureters	Mean Age (y)	Mean Follow-up (mo)	Reflux Resolution (%)	Reported Complications
Peters,[28] 2004	24	27	5.8	—	88 (patients)	Bladder leak and transient voiding dysfunction (1 patient), transient ureteral obstruction (1 patient)
Casale et al,[29] 2008	41	82	3.2	3	97.6 (patients)	Nil
Kasturi et al,[30] 2012	150	300	3.6	3	99.3 (patients)	Nil
Smith et al,[31] 2011	25	33	5.8	16	97 (ureters)	Transient urinary retention (3 patients)
Chalmers et al,[32] 2012	16	22	6.3	11.5	91 (ureters)	Nil
Dangle et al,[33] 2014	29	40	5.4	4	80 (ureters)	Nil
Akhavan et al,[34] 2014	50	78	7.2	10	92 (ureters)	Ureteral obstruction (2 patients), ureteral injury (1 patient), perinephric fluid collection (1 patient), ileus (2 patients), febrile UTI (5 patients), transient urinary retention (1 patient)
Hayashi et al,[35] 2014	7	12	7.6	—	93 (ureters)	Nil
Gundeti et al,[37] 2016	58	83	5.3	30	82 (ureters)	Nil
Grimsby et al,[36] 2015	61	93	6.7	11.7 9	77 (patients)	Ureteral obstruction (3 patients), urine leak (2 patients)
Herz et al,[38] 2016	54	72	5.2	3	85 (ureters)	Transient urinary retention (4 patients)
Boysen et al,[39] 2017	260	363	—	—	88 (ureters)	Transient urinary retention (4 patients)

Abbreviations: UTI, urinary tract infection; VUR, vesicoureteric reflux.

feasibility of the vesicoscopic approach to the bladder was first demonstrated in adults by Gill and colleagues[14] in 2001. In our pilot study using piglets, we have revealed that under carbon dioxide insufflation of the bladder (pneumovesicum) at around 10 mm Hg pressure, a large potential working space could be obtained. This would allow various intravesical procedures, including a Cohen's type of cross-trigonal ureteral reimplantation, or indeed any other intravesical complex reconstruction, to be easily conducted endoscopically using standard laparoscopic instruments. Moreover, we have found that it is physiologically very safe to insufflate the bladder with CO_2 up to 15 mm Hg pressure, with no alteration in renal blood flow or glomerular filtration rates. Subsequently, we reported our initial successful experience with vesicoscopic cross-trigonal ureteral reimplantation under CO_2 insufflation of the bladder in the treatment of dilating primary VUR in infants and children.[13] Our early experience described that endoscopic intravesical ureteral mobilization and cross-trigonal ureteral reimplantation can be safely and effectively performed under CO_2 pneumovesicum with routine laparoscopic surgical techniques and instruments. A high success rate in reflux resolution that was at least equivalent to the open technique, but with much less postoperative pain and bladder spasm, as well as much faster recovery and shorter duration of hospital stay, could be achieved.[13] In addition, results from our center as well as from other workers have revealed no significant late complications on long-term follow-up after pneumovesical ureteral reimplantation.[13,15,16] Valla and colleagues[15] reported their outcome of intravesical ureteral reimplantation under CO_2 pneumovesicum in 72 children with VUR with a success rate of 92%. Kutikov and colleagues[16] reported 32 children who underwent laparoscopic transvesical ureteral reimplantation. Cross-trigonal reimplantation was performed in 27 patients and a Glenn-Anderson reimplantation was performed in 5 patients with primary obstructing megaureter. Success rates were noted to be 92.6% and 80%, respectively. Notwithstanding these early successful reports, the restricted space inside the infant bladder as well as the difficulty to establish and maintain CO_2 pneumovesicum have posed significant technical challenges, thereby limiting the popularity of this technique.[13–16]

With the advent of robotics in the early 2000s, pediatric urologists have been quick to incorporate this technology into the performance of ureteral reimplantation in young children (see **Table 3**). Peters and Woo[17] first reported in 2005 a series of 6 children successfully undergoing robotic-assisted transvesical cross-trigonal ureteral reimplantation. There were no open conversions, and the duration of hospital stay ranged from 2 to 4 days. One patient had a urine leak postoperatively secondary to inadequate port site closure.[17] The authors commented that the robotic-assisted pneumovesicoscopic approach is safe and feasible, with excellent surgical visibility, but could be technically challenging.[17] In a retrospective study, Marchini and colleagues[18] compared 4 cohorts of patients: intravesical open ureteral reimplantation versus intravesical robotic reimplantation, and extravesical open reimplantation versus extravesical robotic reimplantation. The overall success rates ranged from 92% to 100%, which were equivalent between the robotic and the open surgery groups. In the intravesical group, those undergoing robotic ureteral reimplantation had significantly shorter length of hospital stay (43.4 vs 69.6 hours), shorter duration of catheter drainage, and fewer bladder spasms than the open surgery group. However, no such differences were found between the robotic and open extravesical reimplantation groups.[18] Chan and colleagues[19] in 2012 reported their intravesical robotic ureteral reimplantation experience in 3 children, all with high-grade bilateral VUR. There were no reported intraoperative or postoperative complications. All 3 patients showed reflux resolution on postoperative VCUG, and were free from UTI during the follow-up period. Interestingly, apart from the aforementioned initial studies, we have not found other reports on intravesical robotic assisted ureteral reimplantation published in the literature. This may be related to the technical challenge and a steep learning curve that have limited more widespread adoption of the technique by most pediatric urologists. Moreover, the sheer size of the robotic instruments coupled with the very limited working space inside the pediatric bladder posed further technical difficulties for manipulation. In addition, the larger caliber of the robotic camera and instrument arms increased the risk of port site urine leakage, and might result in poorer wound cosmesis when compared with the conventional laparoscopic reimplantation using 3-mm instruments. Future development of smaller and less bulky robotic instruments may help to overcome these limitations and facilitate further adoption of robotic-assisted surgery inside the small bladder in infants and young children, including cross-trigonal ureteral reimplantation as well as other intravesical reconstructive procedures.

Other workers have explored the possibility of laparoscopic ureteral reimplantation with an extravesical approach. Atala, Schimberg, and Mc Dougall their coworkers conducted independent studies in porcine models and demonstrated the feasibility of MIS approach to VUR in early 1990s.[20–22] Ehrlich and colleagues[23] in 1994 published the first clinical study of laparoscopic correction of VUR in 2 patients. This was followed by Janetschek and colleagues,[24] who reported in 1995 MIS correction of VUR in 6 patients, and concluded that laparoscopic Lich-Gregoir antireflux procedure was a complicated operation, which offered no advantage over the conventional procedure. Later, Lakshmanan and Fung[25] described their experience of laparoscopic extravesical ureteral reimplantation in 2000 with refined techniques. During the early 2000s, there were only limited reports on laparoscopic ureteral reimplantation and this operation was in general perceived as a technically demanding and difficult procedure. Although recent studies have demonstrated that a laparoscopic extravesical transperitoneal approach was a safe and effective approach for the correction of VUR with success rates similar to the open technique, there remained some concerns regarding the long operating times and steep learning curves.[26,27] In addition, the extravesical approach is associated with risks of ureteral obstruction, nerve injury, and urinary retention. Urinary retention is especially seen in cases with bilateral VUR. As a result of all these difficulties and concerns, the laparoscopic approach in general still has not gained popularity or a very wide acceptance in most centers.

In sharp contrast with the great difficulties and technical challenges encountered with the use of robotics for antireflux surgery inside the small infant bladder, pediatric urologists have quickly learned the distinct advantages of applying robotics for laparoscopic extravesical Lich-Gregoir ureteral reimplantation. The superb 3-dimensional view of the da Vinci machine together with the remarkable dexterity offered by the endo-wrist technology makes it a perfect tool for various complex laparoscopic procedures that require fine dissection and suturing in the depth of the pelvis with a limited space. This device has greatly facilitated pediatric urologists to jump start, with a shortened learning curve even with technically demanding reconstructive procedures like extravesical ureteral reimplantation. The dexterity of the robotic arms with multiple degrees of freedom of movement together with the endo-wrist capabilities allows surgeons to work much more easily in a deep and small limited space like the infant pelvis, and in addition provides an unprecedented and ergonomically friendly working condition that is impossible to achieve with conventional MIS using standard laparoscopic camera and straight instruments. Surgeons now can work comfortably and do not need to operate in awkward positions for long hours. Because the peritoneal cavity provides much more space for manipulation of the robotic instruments, the laparoscopic extravesical ureteral reimplantation procedure is particularly well-suited for a robotic approach, in contrast with the intravesical approach. Pediatric urologists are quick to capitalize on these advantages of the use of robotics in pelvic reconstructive surgeries in young children and this has led to a sudden spurt of laparoscopic extravesical ureteral reimplantation soon after the introduction of the da Vinci robot in early 2000s.

Initial reports on the feasibility and safety of robotic-assisted extravesical ureteral reimplantation have been very encouraging. Since first described by Peters and colleagues[26] in 2004, the extravesical approach has been widely used as an alternative to open and laparoscopic reimplantation (see **Table 3**). Casale and colleagues[29] reported their experience with robotic extravesical ureteric reimplantation in 41 children with bilateral vesicoureteral reflux. Their operative success rate was 97.6%. There were no reported complications, including postoperative voiding complications. Subsequently, the same group published 2 years of postoperative follow-up results of 150 children with bilateral VUR (> grade 3), who underwent robotic extravesical transperitoneal ureteral reimplantation. Postoperative VCUG revealed VUR resolution in 99.3%. One patient with bilateral grade 5 VUR that was downgraded to unilateral grade 2 VUR was considered to have treatment failure. No patient had postoperative voiding complications or urinary retention when measured by objective voiding parameters and validated questionnaire. The authors concluded that bilateral nerve-sparing robotic-assisted extravesical ureteral reimplantation is associated with similar success rates as the traditional open approaches, with minimal morbidity and no voiding complications after surgery.[30] Smith and colleagues[31] retrospectively reviewed the surgical outcomes of 2 cohorts of 25 patients who underwent robotic extravesical ureteral reimplantation and open cross-trigonal ureteral reimplantation. The overall success rate, defined as no radiographic or clinical evidence of residual reflux, was 97% for robotic-assisted laparoscopy after a mean follow-up of 16 months, compared with 100% for open reimplantation. The operative time was longer in the robotic cohort as compared with that of the open group (3.1 hours vs 2.6 hours, respectively). Moreover, the authors reported that 16% of the patients in the robotic cohort underwent bilateral ureteric reimplantaion experienced transient postoperative urinary retention. Chalmers and colleagues[32] reported the outcome of extravesical ureteral reimplantation in 17 patients (23 ureters). Complete vesicoureteral reflux resolution was observed in 20 ureters (90.9%), VUR downgraded in 1 ureter, and VUR persisted in 1 ureter. No patients required postoperative catheterization at discharge. Dangle and associates reported the outcome of 29 (40 ureters) children, with high-grade VUR (grades 3–5), who have undergone robot-assisted extravesical ureteral reimplantation. Postoperative VCUG revealed complete resolution of VUR in 32 of 40 ureters (80%). Of the remaining refluxing ureters, downgrading of VUR on VCUG was shown in 7 of 8 ureters (87.5%).[33]

Others have also reported on the use of robotic-assisted laparoscopic extravesical ureteral reimplantation as an antireflux procedure in patients with complicated VUR, and with more variable results. Akhavan and colleagues[34] reported the outcomes of extravesical robotic-assisted extravesical ureteral reimplantation in 50 patients. Dysfunctional elimination syndrome was present in 32 (64%). Ten patients (20%) had prior dextranomer/hyaluronic acid injection, and 2 (4%) had prior ureteroneocystostomy on the ipsilateral side. Six among 78 ureters (7.7%) had persistent reflux postoperatively. Complications occurred in 5 patients (10%), including ileus (n = 2), ureteral obstruction (n = 2), ureteral injury (n = 1), and perinephric fluid collection (n = 1). Transient urinary retention occurred in one. In a more recent series, Hayashi and colleagues[35] reported the outcomes of 9 children (15 ureters) who underwent extravesical robotic ureteral reimplantation. VUR resolved in 93% of ureters. There were no postoperative complications. In a published multiinstitutional assessment of the outcomes and complications of robot-assisted laparoscopic extravesical ureteral reimplantation for VUR, a total of 61 patients (93 ureters) with a mean age of 6.7 years underwent the procedure, of which 32 (52%) were bilateral. At a mean follow-up of 11.7 months, VUR persisted in 14 patients (23%), and 6 patients (10%) had major complications, including ureteral obstruction or ureteral leak. Nine patients (11%) were required to undergo reoperation for persistent vesicoureteral reflux or a surgical complication.[36] The authors reported a higher complication rate and a lower success rate for robot-assisted laparoscopic ureteral reimplantation compared with the gold standard of open reimplantation. Gundeti and colleagues[37] reported the outcome of modified extravesical ureteral reimplantaion in 58 patients (83 ureters) with persistent grade 3 to 5 VUR. Owing to technique modifications, there were 3 patient cohorts for comparison. VUR resolved in 82% of ureters, including 8 of 12 ureters (67%), 8 of 11 ureters (73%), and 52 of 60 ureters (87%) for technique modification cohorts 1, 2, and 3, respectively. There were no ureteral complications at a median follow-up of 30 months. In 2016, Herz and colleagues[38] reported the outcomes of extravesical robotic assisted ureteral reimplantation in 54 children (72 ureters). VUR resolved in 85.2% of ureters and complications were reported 11% including ureteral obstruction (7.4%) or ureteral injury (3.7%). Urinary leak from ureteral injury, and urinary obstruction were more common in patients who underwent bilateral reimplantation. Recently, Boysen and colleagues reported the outcome of children who underwent robot-assisted laparoscopic extravesical ureteral reimplantation at 9 academic centers from 2005 to 2014. A total of 260 patients (363 ureters) underwent robot-assisted laparoscopic extravesical ureteral reimplantation for primary vesicoureteral reflux during the study period. Of the 280 ureters with postoperative voiding cystourethrogram or radionuclide cystogram available, VUR resolved in 246 (87.9%). There were 25 complications overall (9.6%). Moreover, 4 patients (3.9%) had transient urinary retention after bilateral reimplantation.[39] Despite earlier claims that, with robotic assistance, one can visualize better and can perform more delicate dissection at the ureteric hiatus, allowing better preservation of pelvic plexus and avoid nerve injuries, there are ongoing concerns regarding an increased rate of urinary retention after robotic bilateral extravesical ureteral reimplantation. Nonetheless, most recent reports have reported rather encouraging results, further establishing that the minimally invasive approach to VUR, especially with robotic assistance, will become the standard preferred approach.

SUMMARY

The minimally invasive ureteral reimplantation is a very attractive and useful tool in the armamentarium for the management of complicate VUR. Subureteric dextranomer/hyaluronic acid injection, laparoscopic extravesical ureteric reimplantation and pneumovesicoscopic intravesical ureteral reimplantation with or without robotic assistance, are established MIS approaches to management of VUR. When used selectively in appropriate cases, these surgical approaches have the potential to deliver the same results of open surgery with all the benefits of minimally invasive surgery. This has greatly obviated the need to remain dependent on expectant conservative approach with long-term antibiotic prophylaxis in the treatment of complicated VUR.

At present, the high cost and the limited availability of robotics at only tertiary centers, as well as the steep learning curve and high technical skill required for laparoscopic surgery, have restricted the accessibility of these MIS approaches. Nevertheless, the techniques of laparoscopic and/or robotic ureteral reimplantation continues to evolve and more data with long-term outcomes are emerging. These will have a significant bearing on the future general adoption of MIS for management of complicated VUR in infants and young children.

REFERENCES

1. Nguyen HT, Herndon CD, Cooper C, et al. The Society for Fetal Urology consensus statement on the evaluation and management of antenatal hydronephrosis. J Pediatr Urol 2010;6(3):212–31.

2. Lee RS, Cendron M, Kinnamon DD, et al. Antenatal hydronephrosis as a predictor of postnatal outcome: a meta-analysis. Pediatrics 2006;118(2):586–93.

3. Hoberman A, Charron M, Hickey RW, et al. Imaging studies after a first febrile urinary tract infection in young children. N Engl J Med 2003;348(3):195–202.

4. Urinary tract infection in children: diagnosis, treatment and long-term management. London: National Collaborating Centre for Women's and Children's Health; 2007.

5. Hansson S, Dhamey M, Sigstrom O, et al. Dimercapto-succinic acid scintigraphy instead of voiding cystourethrography for infants with urinary tract infection. J Urol 2004;172(3):1071–3.

6. Peters CA, Skoog SJ, Arant BS Jr, et al. Summary of the AUA guideline on management of primary vesicoureteral reflux in children. J Urol 2010;184(3):1134–44.

7. Lendvay TS, Sorensen M, Cowan CA, et al. The evolution of vesicoureteral reflux management in the era of dextranomer/hyaluronic acid copolymer: a pediatric health information system database study. J Urol 2006;176(4):1864–7.

8. Herbst KW, Corbett ST, Lendvay TS, et al. Recent trends in the surgical management of primary vesicoureteral reflux in the era of dextranomer/hyaluronic acid. J Urol 2014;191(5):1628–33.

9. Puri P, O'Donnell B. Correction of experimentally produced vesicoureteric reflux in the piglet by intravesical injection of Teflon. Br Med J 1984;289(6436):5–7.

10. Elder JS, Peters CA, Arant BS Jr, et al. Pediatric Vesicoureteral reflux guidelines panel summary report on the management of primary vesicoureteral reflux in children. J Urol 1997;157(5):1846–51.

11. Elder JS, Diaz M, Caldamone AA, et al. Endoscopic therapy for vesicoureteral reflux: a meta-analysis. I. reflux resolution and urinary tract infection. J Urol 2006; 175(2):716–22.

12. Marotte JB, Smith DP. Extravesical ureteral reimplantation for the correction of primary reflux can be done as outpatient procedures. J Urol 2001;165(6):2228–33.

13. Yeung CK, Sihoe JD, Borzi PA. Endoscopic cross-trigonal ureteral reimplantation under carbon dioxide bladder insufflation: a novel technique. J Endourol 2005; 19(3):295–9.

14. Gill S, Ponsky LE, Desai M, et al. Laparoscopic cross-trigonal Cohen ureteroneocystostomy: novel technique. J Urol 2001;166(5):1811–4.

15. Valla JS, Steyaert H, Carfagna L, et al. Place of minimal access ureteral reimplantation in children. J Pediatr Urol 2007;3(supplement 1):S79.

16. Kutikov A, Guzzo TJ, Canter DJ, et al. Initial experience with laparoscopic transvesical ureteral reimplantation at the Children's Hospital of Philadelphia. J Urol 2006;176(5):2222–5.

17. Peters CA, Woo R. Intravesical robotically assisted bilateral ureteral reimplantation. J Endourol 2005;19:618–21.

18. Marchini GS, Hong YK, Minnillo BJ, et al. Robotic assisted laparoscopic ureteral reimplantation in children: case matched comparative study with open surgical approach. J Urol 2011;185(5):1870–5.

19. Chan KW, Lee KH, Tam YH, et al. Early experience in robotic-assisted laparoscopic bilateral intravesical ureteral reimplantation for vesicoureteral reflux in children. J Robot Surg 2012;6(3):259–62.

20. Atala A, Kavoussi LR, Goldstein DS, et al. Laparoscopic correction of vesicoureteral reflux. J Urol 1993;50(2):748–51.

21. Schimberg W, Wacksman J, Rudd R, et al. Laparoscopic correction of vesicoureteral reflux in the pig. J Urol 1994;151(6):1664–7.

22. Mc Dougall EM, Urban DA, Kerbl K, et al. Laparoscopic repair of vesicoureteral reflux utilizing the Lich-Gregoir technique in the pig model. J Urol 1995;153(2): 497–500.

23. Ehrlich RM, Gershman A, Fuchs G. Laparoscopic vesicoureteroplasty in children: initial case reports. Urology 1994;43(2):255–61.

24. Janetschek G, Radmayr C, Bartsch G. Laparoscopic ureteral anti-reflux plasty reimplantation. First clinical experience. Ann Urol 1995;29(2):101–5.

25. Lakshmanan Y, Fung LC. Laparoscopic extravesicular ureteral reimplantation for vesicoureteral reflux: recent technical advances. J Endourol 2000;14(7):589–93.

26. Lopez MI, Varlet F. Laparoscopic extravesical transperitoneal approach following the Lich-Gregoir technique in the treatment of vesicoureteral reflux in children. J Pediatr Surg 2010;45(4):806–10.

27. Riquelme M, Lopez M, Landa S, et al. Laparoscopic extravesical ureteral reimplantation (LEVUR): a multicenter experience with 95 cases. Eur J Pediatr Surg 2013;23(2):143–7.

28. Peters CA. Robotically assisted surgery in pediatric urology. Urol Clin North Am 2004;31(4):743–52.

29. Casale P, Patel RP, Kolon TF. Nerve sparing robotic extravesical ureteral reimplantation. J Urol 2008;179(5):1987–9.

30. Kasturi S, Sehgal SS, Christman MS, et al. Prospective long-term analysis of nerve-sparing extravesical robotic-assisted laparoscopic ureteral reimplantation. Urology 2012;79(3):680–3.

31. Smith RP, Oliver JL, Peters CA. Pediatric robotic extravesical ureteral reimplantation: comparison with open surgery. J Urol 2011;185(5):1876–81.

32. Chalmers D, Herbst K, Kim C. Robotic-assisted laparoscopic extravesical ureteral reimplantation: an initial experience. J Pediatr Urol 2012;8(3):268–71.

33. Dangle PP, Shah A, Gundeti MS. Robot-assisted laparoscopic ureteric reimplantation: extravesical technique. BJU Int 2014;114(4):630–2.

34. Akhavan A, Avery D, Lendvay TS. Robot-assisted extravesical ureteral reimplantation: outcomes and conclusion from 78 ureters. J Pediatr Urol 2014;10(5): 864–8.

35. Hayashi Y, Mizuno K, Kurokawa S, et al. Extravesical robot-assisted laparoscopic ureteral reimplantation for vesicoureteral reflux: initial experience in Japan with the ureteral advancement technique. Int J Urol 2014;21(10):1016–21.

36. Grimsby GM, Dwyer ME, Jacobs MA, et al. Multi-institutional review of outcomes of robot-assisted laparoscopic extravesical ureteral reimplantation. J Urol 2015; 193(5 Suppl):1791–5.

37. Gundeti MS, Boysen WR, Shah A. Robot-assisted laparoscopic extravesical ureteral reimplantation: technique modifications contribute to optimized outcomes. Eur Urol 2016;70(5):818–23.

38. Herz D, Fuchs M, Todd A, et al. Robot-assisted laparoscopic extravesical ureteral reimplant: a critical look at surgical outcomes. J Pediatr Urol 2016;12(6):402.e1-9.
39. Boysen WR, Ellison JS, Kim C, et al. Multi-institutional review of outcomes and complications of robotic-assisted laparoscopic extravesical ureteral reimplantation for the treatment of primary vesicoureteral reflux in children. J Urol 2017; 197(6):1555–61.

Minimally Invasive Neonatal Surgery

Hirschsprung Disease

Atsuyuki Yamataka, MD, PhD*, Go Miyano, MD, PhD,
Masahiro Takeda, MD, PhD

KEYWORDS

- Hirschsprung disease • Laparoscopy • Transanal pull-through • Anorectal line
- Dentate line

KEY POINTS

- Transanal pull-through should be performed with laparoscopic assistance for optimum outcome.
- The anorectal line ensures that the commencement of transanal dissection is identical for all surgeons, providing predictable promising outcome.
- Transanal dissection during transanal pull-through should commence just proximal to the anorectal line, leaving the anorectal line intact.
- Posterior rectal muscle cuff above the anorectal line should be excised totally to prevent postoperative constipation.
- The dentate line is too subjective as a landmark.

 Video content accompanies this article at http://www.perinatology.theclinics. com.

INTRODUCTION: NATURE OF THE PROBLEM

The primary clinical feature of Hirschsprung disease (HD) is obstruction caused by a lack of propagation of peristalsis; this lack of propagation is associated with the absence of ganglion cells in the myenteric and submucosal plexus.[1,2] Most (75%) patients with HD have ganglion cells down to the level of the rectosigmoid colon; the rest have aganglionosis of the descending colon, splenic flexure, or transverse colon.

Disclosure statement: The authors have nothing to disclose.
Department of Pediatric Surgery, Juntendo University School of Medicine, 2-1-1, Hongo, Bunkyo-ku, Tokyo 113-8421, Japan
* Corresponding author.
E-mail address: yama@juntendo.ac.jp

Of all cases of HD, 80% to 90% are symptomatic and diagnosed during the neonatal period.[1,2] Delayed passage of meconium in the newborn, constipation with intermittent diarrhea, a distended abdomen with bilious vomiting, and feeding intolerance with poor weight gain or even weight loss are frequent clinical signs of HD. Diarrhea in HD is always a symptom of enterocolitis.

The incidence of HD is approximately 1 in 5000 live births; Asian children seem to have the highest incidence at almost 3 per 5000 live births. The male-to-female ratio of HD is approximately 4:1.[1,2]

INDICATIONS/CONTRAINDICATIONS FOR MINIMALLY INVASIVE SURGERY IN HIRSCHSPRUNG DISEASE

The goals of surgical management for HD are to remove the aganglionic bowel and reconstruct the intestinal tract by bringing normally innervated bowel down to the anus while preserving sphincter function. Definitive surgery, that is, pull-through, is indicated once a provisional diagnosis of HD is confirmed by suction rectal biopsy. Operative full-thickness biopsy may be required for diagnosis if suction rectal biopsy is inconclusive. Be wary of overzealous suction biopsies, because rectal bleeding is a potential serious complication.

Most centers will opt for minimally invasive surgery (MIS) over conventional open laparotomy for pull-through (COPT) today, performing transanal pull-through (TAPT) with laparoscopic assistance (L-TAPT) or without (pure TAPT). If rectosigmoid dilatation is extreme, an ileostomy or colostomy can be considered preoperatively to reduce the risks for complications, such as stenosis and wound infection or abscess formation at the coloanal anastomosis.

Contraindications to MIS in neonates with HD may include previous abdominal surgery, severe enterocolitis, massive dilatation and elongation of the colon proximal to the aganglionic segment, or any coexisting condition that will deteriorate during pneumoperitoneum.

SURGICAL TECHNIQUE/PROCEDURE

Here we present the L-TAPT procedure we perform routinely at our institution for HD.

Preoperative Planning

Before surgery, surgeons must appreciate the value of the critical importance of planning because success of surgery does not depend on skill alone. The success or failure of a procedure relies on organization. Thus, every surgeon must take as long as necessary to define the diagnosis requiring surgical intervention and study all the anatomic and technical aspects of the planned surgery and possible anomalies that could complicate progress, then prepare a careful plan of attack. Thus, paramount to this is establishing a diagnosis. This requires obtaining a detailed history from the parents, a thorough physical examination, and all necessary investigations (biochemical, diagnostic imaging, and biopsies). The basis of all preoperative planning is to match the desired outcome with what the treating surgeon is capable of providing, both clinically and technically. There is no golden rule. A preoperative plan should list all the steps necessary for a successful outcome and must be explained to the parents so they are fully aware of the risks and complications that may arise.

Preoperative Preparation and Patient Positioning

Preoperatively, all patients without stomas are fed normally until 2 to 3 days before surgery. Parents are asked to perform bowel irrigations with normal saline to decompress the colon until there is no fecal residue forthcoming. For L-TAPT, a patient is admitted 2 days before surgery and is started on intravenous fluid replacement. The patient is allowed to drink only water after admission, and has bowel irrigations twice daily to clean the colon thoroughly. Intensive bowel preparation is mandatory with L-TAPT. Patients older than 12 months, or infants with dilated tortuous proximal colon, require 3 days of bowel preparation instead of the 2 days mentioned previously. If a patient has a stoma, 2 full days are required for preparing the bowel proximal to the stoma, and 1 full day for preparing the bowel distal to the stoma. A nasogastric tube is inserted before surgery to decompress the intestine. An aminoglycoside antibiotic (100 mg/kg per day) is given orally the day before surgery. Broad-spectrum antibiotics, such as ceftazidime (120 mg/kg per day) or isepamicin sulfate (8 mg/kg per day) are given intravenously once the patient is fully anesthetized.[a]

After induction of general endotracheal tube anesthesia, the patient is positioned at the end of the operating table in the supine position. The rectum is suctioned with a rectal tube to make sure that the bowel has no fecal residue. If there is any vague discoloration or indication of insufficient bowel preparation, surgery must be canceled and rescheduled to prevent postoperative complications at the coloanal anastomosis, such as leakage and abscess formation. The patient's body is disinfected. For infants, the trunk and buttocks are prepared extensively, then the legs circumferentially to the tips of the toes, and sterile stockings are placed on both legs. The legs are raised when transanal dissection is commenced. Children older than infants are positioned in the lithotomy position with their legs in stirrups.

The laparoscopic surgeon and the scopist stand on the patient's right side. The scrub nurse stands at the left lower end of the table. A monitor is positioned beyond the patient's feet. The table is placed head-down (reverse Trendelenburg position) for both laparoscopic colorectal dissection and transanal dissection. A urinary catheter is used to decompress the bladder.

Surgical Approach

TAPT is now applied to patients with HD at most centers; however, COPT, although becoming less popular, is still used. TAPT is usually performed with or without laparoscopic assistance for colorectal dissection, and can be performed in combination with laparotomic colorectal dissection. TAPT is performed using the surgical approaches of the Swenson, Soave, and Duhamel procedures.[2]

SURGICAL PROCEDURE

Our L-TAPT is a modification of the classic procedure of Georgeson and colleagues[3] and the procedure of De La Torre-Mondragon and Ortega-Salgado.[4] The most distinct features are the level at which transanal dissection is commenced and the length of the residual rectal muscle cuff.

Step 1: Laparoscopy-Assisted Colon Suction Biopsy

Laparoscopy-assisted colon suction biopsy can be performed in any infant or child of any size with rectosigmoid-type HD, because the sigmoid colon can be mobilized

---

[a] In many areas of the world we do not have the luxury of a 2-day to 3-day bowel preparation. The editor's practice is to start clear liquids a day or two preoperatively at home, along with dilations and/or enemas. We then administer oral antibiotics and give intravenous antibiotics perioperatively.

readily to allow the tip of the suction biopsy device to reach the proposed biopsy site. Fortuitously, 80% of HD cases are rectosigmoid, and laparoscopic-assisted colon suction biopsy is safe, simple, and quick compared with full-thickness biopsy.

The suction biopsy device we use is 170 to 180 mm in length with a tissue-sampling mechanism located 10 to 15 mm from the tip. After identification of the region of caliber change in the colon laparoscopically by a surgeon from the laparoscopy team (laparoscopic surgeon), the suction biopsy device is inserted into the anus by a surgeon from the transanal pull-through team (perineal surgeon) (**Fig. 1**) ensuring that the tissue-sampling mechanism faces anteriorly to allow the laparoscopic surgeon to check for any possible risks for perforation. The device is advanced until it is proximal to the region of caliber change and the perineal surgeon takes biopsies of the mucosa and submucosa under supervision of the laparoscopic surgeon. The laparoscopic surgeon places a metal laparoscopic vessel clip at the biopsy site as a marker. Biopsy specimens are sent for immediate assessment by a pathologist on stand-by. If the result is aganglionic, the biopsy is repeated more proximally. If ganglion cells are present, the colon is pulled-through to the level of the clip transanally, and a coloanal anastomosis is performed. Before the anastomosis is performed, full-thickness biopsies are taken at 12, 3, 6, and 9 o'clock circumferentially at the level of the clipped biopsy site that has been exposed through the anus, to confirm the presence of ganglion cells in the muscle layers of the distal end of the pulled-through colon.

To date, we have had no incidence of perforation during laparoscopic-assisted suction biopsy. Laparoscopic seromuscular biopsy is widely used; however, there may be a risk for perforation if the biopsy is too deep. If perforation does occur, the defect should be closed with several sutures, but this is time-consuming and likely to cause leakage of bowel contents that, although minor, is completely preventable if biopsies are performed using laparoscopy-assisted suction biopsy.

Step 2: Laparoscopic Colorectal Dissection

A 5-mm port is inserted through the umbilicus using an open Hasson technique and pneumoperitoneum is established with carbon dioxide to a pressure of

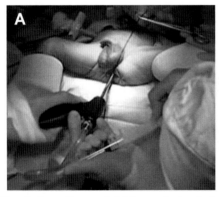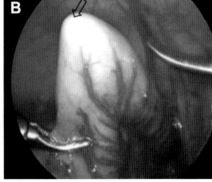

Fig. 1. A suction rectal biopsy device is being advanced (*A*) into the colon through the anus by a surgeon from the transanal pull-through team under supervision of a laparoscopic surgeon until the tip (*B, arrow*) of the device lies proximal to the caliber change.

10 mm Hg. Three additional 3-mm or 5-mm ports are placed in the right upper and lower quadrants, and in the left upper quadrant. A laparoscope is inserted through the 5-mm port in the right upper quadrant. The surgeon's 2 working ports are the umbilical port for the left hand and the right lower abdominal port for the right hand. The port in the left upper abdomen can be used for either retraction of the colon, or, additionally, for the surgeon's left hand.

The operation begins by identifying the level of ganglionic colon using the previously mentioned laparoscopic colon suction biopsy technique or alternative biopsy techniques. If the biopsy site is ganglionic, the laparoscopic surgeon starts dissection of the colorectum. The laparoscopic surgeon or an assistant retracts the distal sigmoid colon toward the anterior abdominal wall with a grasper. Hook diathermy or other energy devices are used for colorectal dissection. Mesenteric vessels are divided distal to the level of the clipped biopsy site, leaving both the marginal artery and vein intact at the level of the clipped biopsy site, which will be the distal end of the pulled-through colon. Then, the mesenteric vascular arcade proximal to the clipped biopsy site is inspected, and a few vessels divided to allow the pulled-through colon to reach the anus without tension; the marginal vessels in the pulled-through colon are thus essentially intact, ensuring good vascular perfusion. Dissection of the colon distal to the clipped biopsy site is performed along the colon wall. Because preserving the marginal vessels is unnecessary, dissection is relatively easy. Further dissection is continued in the rectum distal to the peritoneal reflection circumferentially, which greatly facilitates invagination of the proximal rectum during transanal rectal dissection. The laparoscopic surgeon should identify the location of the ureters and vas deferens (in boys) for dissection of the distal rectum.

A significant advantage of L-TAPT is that the colon can be mobilized keeping the marginal arteries at the distal end of the pull-through colon intact to ensure good blood supply to the coloanal anastomosis. Without laparoscopy, marginal arteries are likely to be injured (**Fig. 2**).

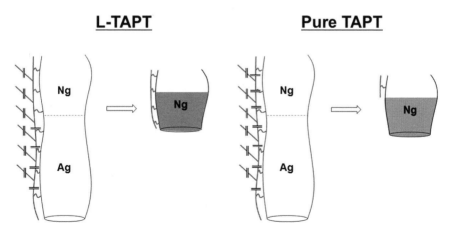

L-TAPT   Pure TAPT

Fig. 2. A significant advantage of L-TAPT is the ability to mobilize the colon while keeping marginal arteries intact, unlike during TAPT without laparoscopic coloanal dissection (pure TAPT) when sacrifice of marginal arteries to the pull-through colon is unavoidable. Short double lines indicate ligation sites. Ag, aganglionic; Ng, normoganglionic.

Step 3: Transanal Dissection

While awaiting histopathology results after laparoscopic colon suction biopsy, the patient is placed in the lithotomy position by flexing the patient's legs and the perineal surgeon places 3 to 0 traction sutures circumferentially 3 to 4 cm from the anus to expose the dentate line (DL). The anal valves along the dentate line at the bottom of the anal sinuses are then hooked up using a Lone Star Ring Retractor System (Lone Star Medical Products, Inc, Stafford, TX), allowing the anorectal line (ARL) to be identified nicely as a ring at the top of the anal columns of Morgagni (**Fig. 3**).[5] The ARL represents the squamous columnar junction of the anal transition zone and is readily visible in viable tissue, but its macroscopic appearance will be lost when tissue is preserved in formalin. By this time, histopathology results should be available. The legs are lowered and, based on biopsy results, further laparoscopic colorectal dissection is performed if required, otherwise, a mesenteric vascular arcade is selected and dissection/mobilization of the ganglionic colon is completed for pull-through.

The patient is again positioned in the lithotomy position by flexing the legs to expose the ARL. Multiple fine traction sutures are placed proximal to the ARL and the mucosa incised just proximal to the ARL circumferentially using needle-tipped electrocautery.

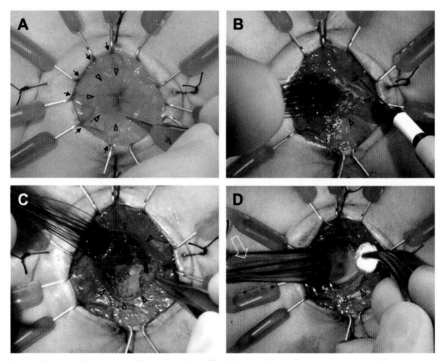

Fig. 3. The ARL (*arrowheads*) can be identified by hooking the crypts (*arrows*) in the DL to expose the anal transitional zone with a ring retractor device (*A*). Note multiple fine traction sutures just proximal to the ARL (*arrowheads*) and incision just proximal to the ARL (*B*), leaving the ARL (*arrowheads*) intact (*C*). A large-bore silicon tube (*large yellow arrow*) has been inserted into the rectal lumen (*D*), which greatly facilitates transanal "submucosal" (an *asterisk*) dissection. Near full-thickness rectal dissection is indicated between the 2 small yellow arrows.

The ARL is left intact (see **Fig. 3**). The perineal surgeon commences near full-thickness rectal dissection transanally progressing cranially for 10 to 15 mm in the plane of the rectal muscle layer (**Fig. 4**), taking great care not to injure the external anal sphincter and levator ani complex, although this is unlikely because transanal dissection is within the plane of the rectal muscles. Nevertheless, dissection should be meticulous. At this stage, a large-bore silicon tube is inserted into the rectal lumen (see **Fig. 3**) and the plane of dissection is changed to the submucosal plane and continued proximally between the rectal mucosa and the rectal muscle layers (see **Fig. 4**). The tube acts as a stent, greatly facilitating submucosal dissection. As mucosectomy progresses further proximally, the devascularized rectosigmoid colon that has already been prepared laparoscopically for pull-through begins to invaginate into the rectal muscle cuff and reaches the anus easily without need for dividing mesenteric vessels transanally. When this invagination starts, submucosal dissection is considered to be sufficient and the invaginated muscular wall of the rectum is divided circumferentially. The proximal rectosigmoid is delivered through the anus externally without applying tension until the proposed site for the coloanal anastomosis marked by the metal clip is identified.

After the proposed site for the coloanal anastomosis, marked by the clip, is exposed through the anus, we assess if there is any tension, and if there is any suggestion of tension, especially on vessels, further laparoscopic dissection/mobilization is required to prevent retraction of the pulled-through colon that may cause anastomotic leakage or pelvic abscess formation. A coloanal anastomosis under tension may also disrupt postoperative bowel function (POBT).

Step 4: Total Excision of the Posterior Aganglionic Rectal Muscle Cuff

Before the coloanal anastomosis, the aganglionic rectal cuff should be excised. The rectal cuff is divided at the 3 and 9 o'clock positions into anterior and posterior cuffs. The posterior rectal cuff is then divided caudally in the midline down to the ARL to ensure complete release of achalasia and excised at the level of the starting point of the transanal rectal dissection, that is, just proximal to the ARL. In other words, the entire posterior aganglionic rectal cuff is removed, with the first 10 to 15 mm of rectal dissection from the ARL being nearly full-thickness. The 10-mm-long to 15-mm-long remnant of aganglionic rectal wall that is of negligible thickness is divided caudally, or excised ideally, to just proximal to the ARL to achieve complete release of achalasia due to the remaining aganglionic rectal wall. Division or excision of this thin 10 to 15 mm of aganglionic rectal wall should be superficial enough not to injure the pelvic floor muscles surrounding the anorectum. The anterior rectal cuff is also excised to where the laparoscopic dissection was performed, usually slightly distal to the peritoneal reflection.

The pull-through colon is anastomosed to just above the ARL using interrupted absorbable sutures (**Fig. 5**).

COMPLICATIONS AND MANAGEMENT

Complications after L-TAPT can be classified as either early (weeks) or late (months to years). Early serious postoperative complications include anastomotic leakage, retraction of the pulled-through colon, abscess formation at the coloanal anastomosis, or pull-through of a transitional segment of colon. Late complications include bowel obstruction, intractable constipation, enterocolitis, incontinence, and anal stenosis/stricture.

In our experience, there were no intraoperative complications or serious early postoperative complications except 1 neonatal case of postoperative obstruction

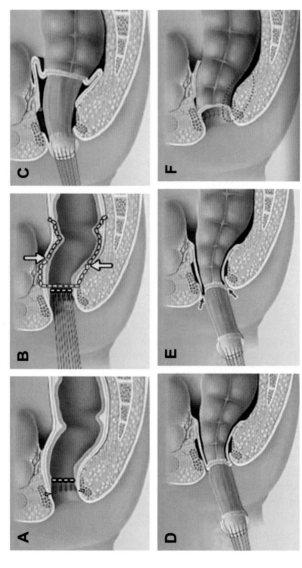

Fig. 4. Anatomic relationships in the anal transitional zone. The DL (*arrowheads*) is at the bottom of the anal sinuses and the ARL (*vertical broken line*) is at the top of the anal columns of Morgagni (*A*). The perineal surgeon commences near full-thickness rectal dissection transanally progressing cranially for 10 to 15 mm in the plane of the rectal muscle layer (*purple broken line*). The yellow arrows indicate where the plane of dissection is changed to submucosal (*B*) and continued proximally between the rectal mucosa and the rectal muscle layers (*maroon broken line*), invaginating the proximal colon to the distal colon (*C*) and finally to the anus (*D*). At this time, the rectal muscle cuff is divided circumferentially (*arrows; E*), the posterior rectal cuff is excised totally (*red dotted circle; F*), and the anterior rectal cuff is excised to where the laparoscopic dissection was performed (*red arrowhead*).

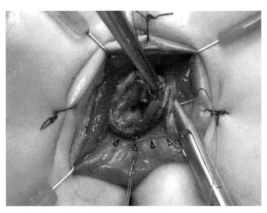

Fig. 5. The pull-through colon (*asterisk*) being anastomosed to the ARL (*arrowheads*) using interrupted sutures.

caused by residual rectal cuffs that had only been split in the midline and had become folded caudally toward the anus outside the pulled-through colon during pull-through of normally innervated colon down to the anus.[6] This patient required redo surgery to remove the residual rectal cuffs using a posterior sagittal approach. Because of this case, we began to excise the posterior rectal cuff in toto because splitting the rectal cuff in the midline may cause obstruction after surgery.

POSTOPERATIVE CARE

Provided L-TAPT is performed meticulously without any complications, unremarkable recovery is to be expected with routine postoperative care. Intravenous fluids and nasogastric decompression are continued postoperatively until bowel function returns. The urinary catheter is left in place until the next morning. As soon as bowel function returns, oral intake is initiated with tapering of intravenous fluids, typically by 3 to 4 days postoperatively. Intravenous antibiotics are continued for 3 days postoperatively and patients can be discharged once a full oral diet is tolerated. Rectal examination is performed 3 to 4 weeks after discharge and anal dilatation commenced if necessary.

OUTCOMES
Assessing Postoperative Bowel Function

We assess POBF based on a standard questionnaire we developed that assesses fecal continence by scoring several parameters (frequency of motions, severity of staining/soiling, severity of perianal erosions, anal shape, requirement for medication) as poor = 0, acceptable = 1, and good = 2; maximum score = 10. Our POBF questionnaire also overcomes a commonly held misconception that continence cannot be evaluated effectively in patients younger than 4 years,[7] and invite surgeons to include our bowel function questionnaire in their routine follow-up of patients with HD after pull-through because it does not include an assessment of urge to defecate, which cannot practically be assessed accurately until the ages of 3 or 4 years. A 7-year comparison of annual POBF scores between L-TAPT and COPT that we reported in 2007 found L-TAPT to have better scores throughout (**Fig. 6**); however, differences were not statistically significant.

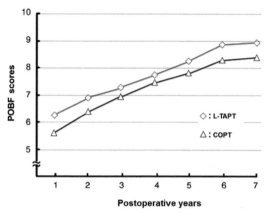

Fig. 6. POBF scores for L-TAPT were consistently better than for COPT, but not statistically significant (*P* = NS).

Midterm Follow-up after Laparoscopic Transanal Pull-Through: Dentate Line Versus Anorectal Line

We recently conducted a midterm prospective comparison of postoperative outcomes between DL and ARL patients after changing to using the ARL during L-TAPT in 2007. For thoroughness, we added sensation of rectal fullness and ability to distinguish flatus from stool (as poor = 0, acceptable = 1, and good = 2) to the previously reported POBF questionnaire to give a maximum score of 14. There were 2 cases of colitis in both ARL (6.1%) and DL (4.9%) (*P* = NS); all were treated successfully as outpatients by colonic decompression and intravenous antibiotics. None of our subjects had constipation. Mean annual POBF scores from 4 to 7 years postoperatively were 9.7 ± 1.9 (*P*<.05), 10.1 ± 1.6 (*P*<.05), 10.6 ± 1.6, and 11.3 ± 1.4 (*P*<.05) in ARL and 8.6 ± 1.5, 9.1 ± 1.9, 9.8 ± 1.9, 10.0 ± 1.6 in DL (**Fig. 7**). Maximum duration of follow-up after L-TAPT using the ARL was 8 years in our last report in 2015,[8] and further follow-up would suggest that outcome continues to be excellent, indicating that L-TAPT using the ARL is the procedure of choice for treating HD. We believe the low incidence of postoperative constipation in our series is because of the total

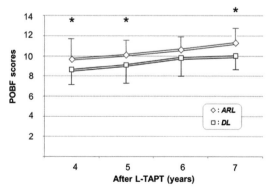

Fig. 7. Change in mean POBF scores over time. Mean annual POBF scores at 4, 5, and 7 years were significantly better when the ARL was used instead of the DL (**P*<.05).

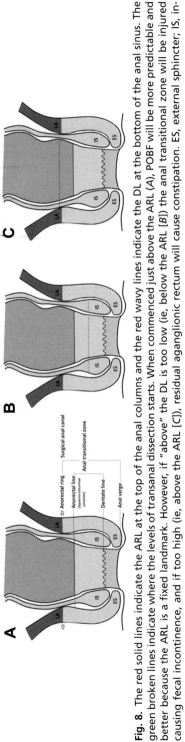

Fig. 8. The red solid lines indicate the ARL at the top of the anal columns and the red wavy lines indicate the DL at the bottom of the anal sinus. The green broken lines indicate where the levels of transanal dissection starts. When commenced just above the ARL (A), POBF will be more predictable and better because the ARL is a fixed landmark. However, if "above" the DL is too low (ie, below the ARL [B]) the anal transitional zone will be injured causing fecal incontinence, and if too high (ie, above the ARL [C]), residual aganglionic rectum will cause constipation. ES, external sphincter; IS, internal sphincter; LA, levator ani.

excision of the posterior rectal cuff caudally, almost down to the ARL, that we now perform routinely.

SUMMARY

The DL is the traditional landmark for dissection, yet distances ranging from 5 to 20 mm[1,9] have been reported to be appropriate even though it is well known that if commenced too high, there is a tendency for constipation, and if commenced too low, there is a tendency for staining (**Fig. 8**). The distance chosen above the DL would appear to be quite subjective, especially when the age and physique of a patient are also taken into account, with the result that postoperative outcome in patients in whom the DL is used as a landmark can be somewhat unpredictable. The ARL is a reproducibly recognizable landmark without any need for subjective interpretation (see **Fig. 8**) in contrast to "above" the DL.

With our L-TAPT technique using the ARL,[8] the anal transitional zone between the DL and the ARL is preserved, ensuring that the anorectum has normal sensory and motor function, minimizing postoperative fecal staining/soiling. In fact, in our most recent research using HD model mice, we found there appears to be no difference in sensory innervation anal transitional zone, compared with normal mice,[10] proof of the importance of an intact anal transitional zone.

There are also reports about short residual cuff remnants not being associated with POBF sequelae in pure TAPT without laparoscopic assistance and L-TAPT cases,[11] but we do not recommend leaving any aganglionic cuff, let alone a short one, because there may be a subgroup of patients in whom the balance of peristalsis in the pull-through colon cannot overcome the achalasia in the cuff remnant and cause some degree of residual constipation that would otherwise not be an issue if there was no cuff. We believe that the good POBF results achieved in our L-TAPT cases are due entirely to total excision of the posterior cuff above the ARL and transanal dissection starting just above the ARL. We wonder if the increasing number of reports of poor POBF after TAPT with or without laparoscopy may be in cases with cuff remnants and/or in whom the level of transanal dissection was based on the DL rather than the ARL.

Our experience would indicate that L-TAPT using the ARL preserves innervation of the anal transitional zone and laparoscopic assistance improves mobilization of the pulled-through colon (Video 1). Although some investigators[12–15] have very recently reported what we believe to be are disappointing outcomes after TAPT with or without laparoscopic assistance, including POBF, we are confident that if our technique is used by surgeons with a sound knowledge of anatomic relationships in the anal transition zone, the resulting outcome will greatly improve.

Best Practices

What is the current practice?

TAPT based on the DL, unpredictable POBF.

Best practice/guideline/care path objective(s)

Efforts to improve/enhance the quality of surgery for HD include laparoscopic assistance and using the ARL instead of the DL. Patient safety and parental satisfaction are promoted. Meticulous dissection with laparoscopic assistance optimizes resources by ensuring the coloanal anastomosis has viable vascularity, and using the ARL as the landmark for dissection ensures good POBF that improves quality of life.

What changes in current practice are likely to improve outcomes?

Abandon DL as the landmark for dissection/excision and use the ARL.

Is there a clinical algorithm?

No. The only major treatment decisions concern histopathology. Is HD proven by biopsy findings and is the potential pull-through bowel ganglionic. The following are the key points of our L-TAPT procedure.
- Biopsy-proven diagnosis (preferably laparoscopic suction rectal biopsy)
- L-TAPT for preserving the marginal vessels in the pull-through colon
- ARL-based dissection
- Excision of all cuffs to eliminate achalasia due to residual aganglionic rectal wall
- Objective assessment of POBF immediately after surgery, then at least annually

Major recommendations

Use the ARL and laparoscopic assistance.

Clinical algorithm(s)

Suspected HD→ Biopsy→ If HD→ Primary L-TAPT or if the patient has a tortuous proximal colon with extreme dilatation, or is older (than 12 months) a colostomy is created followed by L-TAPT as a secondary procedure. If HD cannot be diagnosed on biopsy, close follow-up and management of constipation and/or abdominal distension and further investigations to exclude other disorders of bowel motility, such as allied HD.

Rating for the strength of the evidence

We consider the rating for the recommendations we presented is of the highest strength; that is, recommendations are based on consistent and good-quality patient-orientated evidence.

Bibliographic source

In the preparation of this article, the listed references were combined with personal experiences to describe our L-TAPT procedure.

Summary statement

Good POBF can be expected with L-TAPT using the ARL because the anal transitional zone is preserved and the ARL is intact. Laparoscopic dissection of the colorectum also preserves the marginal vessels in the pulled-through colon, ensuring a reliable coloanal anastomosis.

SUPPLEMENTARY DATA

Supplementary data related to this article can be found online at http://dx.doi.org/10.1016/j.clp.2017.08.006.

REFERENCES

1. Puri P. Hirschsprung's disease. In: Puri P, editor. Newborn surgery. London: Arnold; 2003. p. 513–33.
2. Langer JC. Hirschsprung disease. In: Holcomb GW 3rd, Murphy JP, Ostlie DJ, editors. Ashcraft's pediatric surgery. 6th edition. Philadelphia: Saunders Elsevier; 2010. p. 474–91.
3. Georgeson KE, Fuenfer MM, Hardin WD. Primary laparoscopic pull-through for Hirschsprung's disease in infants and children. J Pediatr Surg 1995;30:1017–22.
4. De la Torre-Mondragon L, Ortega-Salgado JA. Transanal endorectal pull-through for Hirschsprung's disease. J Pediatr Surg 1998;33(8):1283–6.
5. Finger C. Histology of the anal canal. Am J Surg Pathol 1988;12(1):41–55.

6. Shimotakahara A, Yamataka A, Kobayashi H, et al. Obstruction due to rectal cuff after laparoscopy-assisted transanal endorectal pull-through for Hirschsprung's disease. J Laparoendosc Adv Surg Tech A 2006;16(5):540–2.

7. Yamataka A, Kaneyama K, Fujiwara N, et al. Rectal mucosal dissection during transanal pull-through for Hirschsprung's disease: the anorectal or the dentate line? J Pediatr Surg 2009;44(1):266–9.

8. Miyano G, Koga H, Okawada M, et al. Rectal mucosal dissection commencing directly on the anorectal line versus commencing above the dentate line in laparoscopy-assisted transanal pull-through for Hirschsprung's disease: prospective medium-term follow-up. J Pediatr Surg 2015;50:2041–3.

9. Bischoff A, Frischer J, Knod JL, et al. Damaged anal canal as a cause of fecal incontinence after surgical repair for Hirschsprung disease—a preventable and under-reported complication. J Pediatr Surg 2017;52(4):549–53.

10. Takeda M, Miyahara K, Akazawa C, et al. Sensory innervation of the anal canal and anorectal line in Hirschsprung's disease. Histological evidence from mouse models. Pediatr Surg Int 2017;33(8):883–6.

11. Nasr A, Langer JC. Evolution of the technique in the transanal pull-through for Hirschsprung's disease: effect on outcome. J Pediatr Surg 2007;42(1):36–40.

12. Neuvonen MI, Kyrklund K, Rintala RI, et al. Bowel function and quality of life after transanal endorectal pull-through for Hirschsprung disease: controlled outcomes up to adulthood. Ann Surg 2017;265:622–9.

13. Onishi S, Nakane K, Yamada K, et al. Long-term outcome of bowel function for consecutive cases of Hirschsprung's disease: comparison of the abdominal approach with transanal approach more than 30 years in a single institution—is the transanal approach truly beneficial for bowel function? J Pediatr Surg 2016;51(12):2010–4.

14. Bjornland K, Pakarinen MP, Stenstrom P, et al. A Nordic multicenter survey of long-term bowel function after transanal endorectal pull-through in 200 patients with rectosigmoid Hirschsprung disease. J Pediatr Surg 2017;52(9):1458–64.

15. Neuvonen MI, Kyrklund K, Lindahl HG, et al. A population-based, complete follow-up of 146 consecutive patients after transanal mucosectomy for Hirschsprung disease. J Pediatr Surg 2015;50(10):1653–8.

Inguinal Hernia

Sophia Abdulhai, MD, Ian C. Glenn, MD, Todd A. Ponsky, MD*

KEYWORDS

- Inguinal hernia • Laparoscopic herniorrhaphy • Incarcerated inguinal hernia
- Hydrodissection • Patent processus vaginalis

KEY POINTS

- The incidence of a patent processus vaginalis (or canal of Nuck in females) is highest in premature infants, and many of them close before 2 years of age.
- Not all patent processus vaginalis will develop into a clinical hernia.
- The optimal time of repair for premature and low birth weight infants is controversial.
- Laparoscopy is a safe and possibly technically easier technique, especially for incarcerated inguinal hernias.
- Recurrence rates are reported between 0.4% and 4.1%, but the recurrence rates are decreasing with increasing surgeon experience and are now comparable with open repair.

INTRODUCTION

Inguinal hernias are one of the most common congenital anomalies seen by pediatric surgeons. The overall incidence ranges from 0.8% to 5.0% in full-term infants and up to 30.0% in low birth weight and premature infants.[1–3]

Although open repair is still widely performed, laparoscopic repair is now known to be a safe and effective alternative, with postoperative complication rates comparable with open repair.[4,5] Given the minimal dissection required, especially in complex hernia repairs (ie, incarcerated, recurrent, obese patients), laparoscopy has also been reported by some surgeons to be technically easier.[4,6–9] Laparoscopy may also result in a shorter hospital stay, decreased postoperative pain, and better cosmesis.[9,10] Additionally, laparoscopy also allows for contralateral evaluation and repair of a patent processus vaginalis (PPV) without the need of an additional incision.[11,12]

INDICATIONS/CONTRAINDICATIONS
Clinical Presentation

Most inguinal hernias are found incidentally by a parent or during a routine medical examination. Inguinal hernias present as an intermittent groin bulge that most often

Disclosures: CONMED Advisory Board Member (T A. Ponsky).
Division of Pediatric Surgery, Akron Children's Hospital, One Perkins Square, Suite 8400, Akron, OH 44308, USA
* Corresponding author.
E-mail address: tponsky@chmca.org

occurs when patients bear down. If the hernia is incarcerated, it will present as an irreducible bulge that is not fluctuant but possibly erythematous. Patients may also have obstructive symptoms, such as nausea/vomiting, abdominal distention, and obstipation. Strangulated hernias may also present with peritonitis, bloody stools, and hemodynamic changes.

Premature/Low Birth Weight Infants

There is currently no clear consensus as to the optimal time for herniorrhaphy in premature and low birth weight infants. The argument is that although premature and low birth weight infants are at a high risk of incarceration and infarction,[13,14] they are also at a high risk of anesthesia-related postoperative cardiopulmonary complications, particularly apnea and bradycardia.[15]

Vaos and colleagues[16] recommend early elective herniorrhaphy in premature infants given the high risk of incarceration and postoperative complications; however, Lee and colleagues[17] found the risk of incarceration in their patient population to be low and herniorrhaphy before discharge from the neonatal intensive care unit (NICU) was associated with a prolonged hospital stay. A survey of pediatric surgeons in the United States found that most (63%) will operate before discharge from the NICU.[18]

Timing of Surgery

Although there is concern about the effects of early anesthetic exposure on neurodevelopment,[19] it is recommended that all patients with an inguinal hernia undergo a repair shortly after diagnosis given the risk of incarceration. Stylianos and colleagues[13] found that up to 35% of their patients who presented with an incarcerated hernia were known to have an asymptomatic inguinal hernia. Additionally, the risk of complications, such as infections, recurrence, and testicular atrophy, are increased in incarcerated hernias compared with elective repairs.[13,20,21]

Contraindications

The pneumoperitoneum used during laparoscopy may result in multiple physiologic changes secondary to increased intra-abdominal pressure, such as decreased cardiac filling, reduced functional residual capacity, and increased intracranial pressure.[22,23] It should be used with caution in patients with cardiopulmonary and neurologic issues. Other potential contraindications to laparoscopy include coagulopathies, multiple previous abdominal surgeries, or hemodynamic instability (**Table 1**).

SURGICAL TECHNIQUE/PROCEDURE
Anatomy

Most pediatric inguinal hernias are indirect, resulting from failure of the processus vaginalis (or canal of Nuck in females) to obliterate during fetal development. The

Table 1 Contraindications to laparoscopy	
Relative Contraindications to Laparoscopy	**Absolute Contraindication to Laparoscopy**
Coagulopathies	Hemodynamic instability
Previous abdominal surgery	
Increased intracranial pressure	
Cardiopulmonary disorders	

incidence is higher in premature infants, as the PPV normally closes between 36 and 40 weeks of gestation.

The deep internal ring transmits the spermatic cord in males and the round ligament in females through the inguinal canal. The inferior epigastric vessels are anteromedial to the internal ring; the spermatic vessels run through the lateral/inferior aspect of the internal ring, and the vas deferens passes through the inferior/medial aspect of the internal ring (**Fig. 1**). It is critical to stay superficial, just deep to the peritoneum, when placing the stitch to avoid the spermatic cord and the genital branch of the genitofemoral nerve, which enters the internal ring inferior/lateral adjacent to the spermatic vessels.

Preoperative Planning

Laparoscopic repair is performed under general anesthesia. Routine preoperative antibiotics are not generally given for elective inguinal hernia repairs, but they should be considered for incarcerated hernias given the higher risk of wound infections. Patients should void before the procedure to obviate a urinary catheter. The bladder can also be emptied after anesthesia using the Credé maneuver.

Prep and Patient Positioning

Patients should be placed in the supine position. The Trendelenburg position may facilitate visualization of the pelvis by displacing the bowel caudally. The scrotum should be prepped in addition to the abdomen. This prep will allow the surgeon to push on the scrotum to remove pneumoperitoneum before ligation of the hernia sac.

The operating surgeon may stand on the ipsilateral side of the hernia, but the authors prefer to always stand on patients' left side. The assistant stands on the same side as the surgeon, closer to the head of patients. The monitor should be at the foot of the bed.

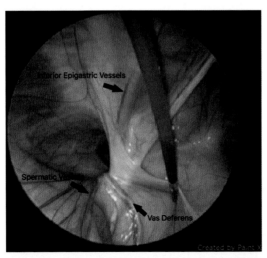

Fig. 1. This image is of a left-sided inguinal hernia. The inferior epigastric vessels are seen superiorly. The peritoneum is pulled back by the Maryland; the spermatic vessels are to the inferior/lateral of the internal ring, and the vas deferens is inferior/medial.

Surgical Approach

There are multiple laparoscopic inguinal herniorrhaphy techniques, using either an intraperitoneal or extraperitoneal approach. The authors focus on a 2-port extraperitoneal approach, which is a variation of the percutaneous internal ring suturing (PIRS) technique.[24,25] This technique involves percutaneous placement of a suture around the internal ring like the PIRS technique but with the addition of hydrodissection and placement of an additional stab incision for an instrument to cause thermal injury to the peritoneum. Thermal injury is performed to create scar tissue, which was found to increase the strength of the closure in a rabbit model.[26]

The equipment used is a single laparoscope (70°/3-mm in neonates, 30°/5-mm in larger children), Maryland dissector or hook cautery, 18-gauge spinal needle, 3-0 monofilament suture, 2-0 permanent braided suture, and a 25-gauge finder needle.[24]

Surgical Procedure

- The 18-gauge needle is first bent, using 2 needle drivers, to create a curve. The 3-0 monofilament suture is folded in half and the looped end is threaded through the 18-gauge needle, with the end just inside the tip of the needle (**Fig. 2**).
- The laparoscope is placed through an infraumbilical trocar once the desired pneumoperitoneum is reached.
- The 3-mm Maryland dissector or hook cautery is placed through a stab incision in the lower abdomen, either in the left lower abdomen (authors' preference) or on the ipsilateral side of the hernia.
- The Maryland dissector or hook cautery is used to cauterize the peritoneum around the internal ring, from the 8- to 5-o'clock position avoiding the spermatic vessels and vas deferens (**Fig. 3**).
- A 25-gauge finder needle is used to identify the 12-o'clock position of the internal ring. A 1-mm incision is made just anterior to this, which is where the spinal needle will be placed.
- The finder needle is placed just anterior to the peritoneum, and hydrodissection is performed using a long-acting local anesthetic to dissect the peritoneum away from the cord structures (**Fig. 4**).
- The spinal needle is then placed through the incision and then inserted until it can be seen beneath the peritoneum at the 12-o'clock position.

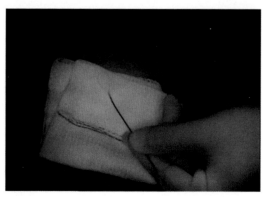

Fig. 2. The 18-gauge spinal needle is bent; the 3-0 monofilament is folded in half, and the looped end is threaded through the needle.

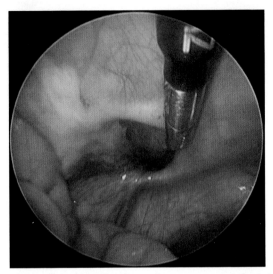

Fig. 3. The Maryland is used to cauterize the peritoneum around the internal ring.

- It is then passed around the internal ring laterally in the hydrodissection plane.
- The needle is placed over the spermatic vessels and vas deferens, if possible. The 3-mm Maryland may be used to assist lifting the peritoneum off the cord structures to allow for safer passage of the needle (**Fig. 5**).
- After passing the vessels, the needle tip should pierce through the peritoneum, around the 6-o'clock position. The loop of the monofilament suture is then pushed out of the needle, and the needle is removed leaving the suture in place (**Fig. 6**).

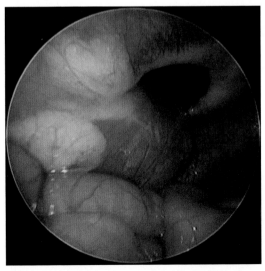

Fig. 4. A 25-gauge finder needle is used to perform hydrodissection using a long-acting local anesthetic between the peritoneum and posterior abdominal wall.

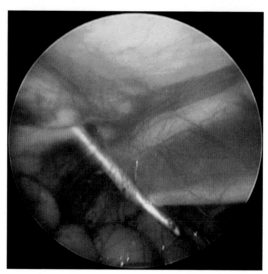

Fig. 5. The spinal needle is then passed around the internal ring laterally in the hydrodissection plane. After passing the vessels, the needle tip is pushed through the peritoneum.

- The needle is then placed medially to the internal ring, again with a folded monofilament suture and again passed through the hydrodissected plane just as previously described from the 12-o'clock position to just lateral to the vas deferens at the location of the first suture. If the vas deferens is difficult to pass over, then the needle can be pierced through the peritoneum just medial to the vas deferens leaving that bit of peritoneum in place.
- The needle is then placed through the first loop, and the first loop is pulled snug against the needle. The second loop is then pushed out of the needle; the needle is removed, allowing the first loop to snugly secure the second loop (**Figs. 7**

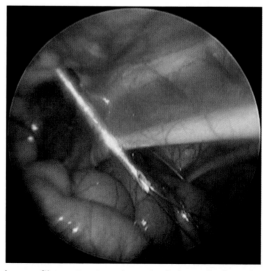

Fig. 6. The looped monofilament suture is pushed through the spinal needle into the pneumoperitoneum.

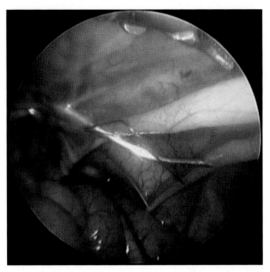

Fig. 7. The spinal needle is then passed around the internal ring medially and then pushed.

and **8**). This first loop is now a snare that can be used to pull the second loop through the lateral edge of the internal ring, allowing the second loop to circumferentially encompass the defect.

- The monofilament suture is then exchanged for a braided, nonabsorbable suture. This exchange is performed by looping the braided suture around the monofilament loop and then using the monofilament suture to pull the braided suture through.
- The looped portion of the braided suture is then cut. Pressure is applied to the scrotum externally to evacuate any air. The 4 ends of the suture are tied to each other to create 2 knots, resulting in a double ligation (**Fig. 9**). In infants,

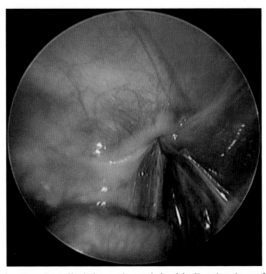

Fig. 8. The braided suture is pulled through, and double ligation is performed.

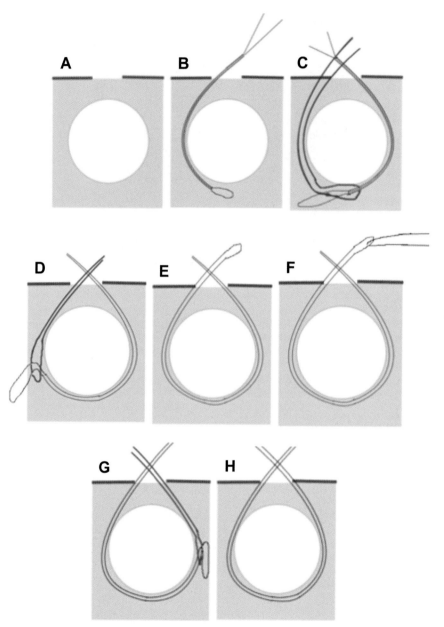

Fig. 9. (*A*) The internal ring. (*B*) The spinal needle being advanced laterally around the internal ring. The looped monofilament suture is then pushed out of the needle. In (*C*), the spinal needle is then advanced medially and pushed through the previous loop. In (*D*), the first loop is placed snugly around the second loop creating a lasso that can be used to pull the second loop circumferentially around the internal ring. (*E*) The second loop of the monofilament suture around the internal ring. The braided suture is looped around the monofilament suture (*F*) and then pulled around the internal ring by the monofilament suture (*G*). The braided suture is now around the internal ring, and double ligation may be performed (*H*).

consider performing single ligation by removing one of the sutures to prevent a suture granuloma.

Alternative Techniques

Extraperitoneal

Single-port techniques and 2-port techniques are both widely used.[27,28] Examples of a single-port technique are the subcutaneous endoscopically assisted ligation (SEAL) and PIRS technique. SEAL involves the placement of a suture percutaneously; then under direct laparoscopic visualization, the suture needle is advanced circumferentially around the internal ring avoiding the cord structures.[29] The PIRS technique uses a spinal needle to encompass the internal ring.[25]

Intraperitoneal

This technique is performed using 2 trocars in addition to a camera port. The high ligation and closure of the internal ring is performed intracorporeally using different suturing techniques, such as a purse-string suture, interrupted suture, and Z-stitch.[27,30,31] Endo-looping should only be used in females given the risk of injury to cord structures.[32] The flip-flap hernioplasty is performed by rotating a peritoneal flap medially to cover the inguinal ring and suturing it down.[33]

Resection of the hernia sac without suture ligation has also been described in patients with inguinal ring diameters less than 1 cm, because it is thought that peritoneal scarring will result in inadequate closure of the inguinal ring.[34]

CONSIDERATIONS
Contralateral Repair

The incidence of a contralateral patent processus vaginalis is 8.8% to 33.0%, with the highest incidence in premature infants.[2,35–38] Routine open contralateral explorations are not recommended because the risks associated with an additional incision and open repair outweighs the risk of developing a contralateral hernia.[39–42] However, routine laparoscopic exploration and repair is still controversial. Although laparoscopy, both transumbilical and transinguinal, is considered a safe and effective method of evaluating for a contralateral PPV or hernia, it is unknown if the risk of performing a repair is less than the risk of leaving a PPV, as not all PPVs will be become clinical hernias.[36,43,44] Although contralateral laparoscopic exploration has been found to be cost-effective,[45] PPV has a poor positive predictive value for development of clinical hernias.[46] Burd and colleagues[47] reported that observation has a lower risk of morbidity compared with contralateral exploration.

At this time, the decision is at the discretion of the surgeon and the patients' families and also should be considered in patients at a higher risk of developing an incarcerated hernia (ie, premature infants) or in those who are a high anesthesia risk (ie, patients with cardiopulmonary issues).

Incarcerated Hernia

Nonoperative reduction is successful in more than 80% of cases and should be attempted in infants unless there is concern for bowel compromise.[13,48] Emergent operative intervention should be performed if there is concern of an incomplete reduction. Repair of the hernia should be performed during the same admission given the high risk of reincarceration.[20]

Laparoscopy is now considered a safe approach to repair of incarcerated hernias, and it also considered technically easier than open surgery.[6,7,49] Advantages are the ability to bypass edematous tissue, avoid cord structures, perform reduction under visual inspection, and inspect the incarcerated organ at the end of the procedure. It also allows for easier reduction because of mechanical widening of the internal ring from the pneumoperitoneum.[6,7]

COMPLICATIONS AND MANAGEMENT

The overall risk of perioperative complications for an elective laparoscopic hernia repair is 0.6% to 1.2%.[21,35,50–52] Potential perioperative complications include testicular or ovarian atrophy, hydrocele, surgical site infection, and injury to surrounding structures, such as cord structures and the bladder. The risk increases significantly with incarcerated hernias, reported between 4.5% and 33.0%.[13,20]

POSTOPERATIVE CARE

Close monitoring in the NICU should be considered for premature and low birth weight infants.[15] Most patients are discharged home by postoperative day 1 for elective laparoscopic hernia repair.

OUTCOMES

The risk of recurrence is reported between 0.4% and 4.1%,[4,9,28,51,53] with the incidence decreasing with time likely from increasing experience. Chan and colleagues[53] found in a retrospective review of 451 laparoscopic inguinal hernia repairs that creating some technical modifications, such as hydrodissection to prevent tension on their purse-string suture, reduced their risk of recurrence from 4.88% to 0.4%.

SUMMARY

Laparoscopy is a safe and effective technique in treating inguinal hernias, including in premature and low birth weight infants and in incarcerated hernias. There are multiple laparoscopic inguinal herniorrhaphy approaches, such as single- and 2-port extraperitoneal techniques and completely intraperitoneal techniques. The authors' extraperitoneal technique described in this article includes hydrodissection, thermal injury to the peritoneum on the inguinal ring, and double ligation of the internal ring. The overall complication and recurrence rates of laparoscopic inguinal hernia repairs are comparable with open repair.

REFERENCES

1. Chang S-J, Chen JY-C, Hsu C-K, et al. The incidence of inguinal hernia and associated risk factors of incarceration in pediatric inguinal hernia: a nation-wide longitudinal population-based study. Hernia 2016;20(4):559–63.
2. Burgmeier C, Dreyhaupt J, Schier F. Comparison of inguinal hernia and asymptomatic patent processus vaginalis in term and preterm infants. J Pediatr Surg 2014;49(9):1416–8.
3. Lautz TB, Raval MV, Reynolds M. Does timing matter? A national perspective on the risk of incarceration in premature neonates with inguinal hernia. J Pediatr 2011;158(4):573–7.
4. Schier F. Laparoscopic inguinal hernia repair—a prospective personal series of 542 children. J Pediatr Surg 2006;41(6):1081–4.
5. Ponsky TA, Nalugo M, Ostlie DJ. Pediatric laparoscopic inguinal hernia repair: a review of the current evidence. J Laparoendosc Adv Surg Tech 2014;24(3): 183–7.

6. Kaya M, Hückstedt T, Schier F. Laparoscopic approach to incarcerated inguinal hernia in children. J Pediatr Surg 2006;41(3):567–9.

7. Esposito C, Turial S, Alicchio F, et al. Laparoscopic repair of incarcerated inguinal hernia. A safe and effective procedure to adopt in children. Hernia 2013;17(2): 235–9.

8. Dutta S, Albanese C. Transcutaneous laparoscopic hernia repair in children: a prospective review of 275 hernia repairs with minimum 2-year follow-up. Surg Endosc 2009;23(1):103–7.

9. Parelkar SV, Oak S, Gupta R, et al. Laparoscopic inguinal hernia repair in the pediatric age group—experience with 437 children. J Pediatr Surg 2010;45(4): 789–92.

10. Zhou X, Peng L, Sha Y, et al. Transumbilical endoscopic surgery for incarcerated inguinal hernias in infants and children. J Pediatr Surg 2014;49(1):214–7.

11. Geisler DP, Jegathesan S, Parmley MC, et al. Laparoscopic exploration for the clinically undetected hernia in infancy and childhood. Am J Surg 2001;182(6): 693–6.

12. Bhatia AM, Gow KW, Heiss KF, et al. Is the use of laparoscopy to determine presence of contralateral patent processus vaginalis justified in children greater than 2 years of age? J Pediatr Surg 2004;39(5):778–81.

13. Stylianos S, Jacir NN, Harris BH. Incarceration of inguinal hernia in infants prior to elective repair. J Pediatr Surg 1993;28(4):582–3.

14. Rajput A, Gauderer MWL, Hack M. Inguinal hernias in very low birth weight infants: incidence and timing of repair. J Pediatr Surg 1992;27(10):1322–4.

15. Murphy JJ, Swanson T, Ansermino M, et al. The frequency of apneas in premature infants after inguinal hernia repair: do they need overnight monitoring in the intensive care unit? J Pediatr Surg 2008;43(5):865–8.

16. Vaos G, Gardikis S, Kambouri K, et al. Optimal timing for repair of an inguinal hernia in premature infants. Pediatr Surg Int 2010;26(4):379–85.

17. Lee SL, Gleason JM, Sydorak RM. A critical review of premature infants with inguinal hernias: optimal timing of repair, incarceration risk, and postoperative apnea. J Pediatr Surg 2011;46(1):217–20.

18. Antonoff MB, Kreykes NS, Saltzman DA, et al. American Academy of Pediatrics section on surgery hernia survey revisited. J Pediatr Surg 2005;40(6):1009–14.

19. Davidson A, Flick RP. Neurodevelopmental implications of the use of sedation and analgesia in neonates. Clin Perinatol 2013;40(3):559–73.

20. Niedzielski J, Kr IR, Gawłowska A. Could incarceration of inguinal hernia in children be prevented? Med Sci Monit 2003;9(1):CR16–8.

21. Rescorla FJ, Grosfeld JL. Inguinal hernia repair in the perinatal period and early infancy: clinical considerations. J Pediatr Surg 1984;19(6):832–7.

22. Nwokoma NJ, Tsang T. Laparoscopy in children and infants. In: Shamsa A, editor. Advanced laparoscopy. InTech; 2011. Available at: http://www.intechopen.com/books/advanced-laparoscopy/laparoscopy-in-children-and-infants. Accessed September 12, 2017.

23. Kalfa N. Tolerance of laparoscopy and thoracoscopy in neonates. Pediatrics 2005;116(6):e785–91.

24. Ostlie DJ, Ponsky TA. Technical options of the laparoscopic pediatric inguinal hernia repair. J Laparoendosc Adv Surg Tech 2014;24(3):194–8.

25. Patkowski D, Czernik J, Chrzan R, et al. Percutaneous internal ring suturing: a simple minimally invasive technique for inguinal hernia repair in children. J Laparoendosc Adv Surg Tech 2006;16(5):513–7.

26. Blatnik JA, Harth KC, Krpata DM, et al. Stitch versus scar—evaluation of laparo-scopic pediatric inguinal hernia repair: a pilot study in a rabbit model. J Laparoendosc Adv Surg Tech 2012;22(8):848–51.

27. Saranga Bharathi R, Arora M, Baskaran V. Minimal access surgery of pediatric inguinal hernias: a review. Surg Endosc 2008;22(8):1751–62.

28. Takehara H, Yakabe S, Kameoka K. Laparoscopic percutaneous extraperitoneal closure for inguinal hernia in children: clinical outcome of 972 repairs done in 3 pediatric surgical institutions. J Pediatr Surg 2006;41(12):1999–2003.

29. Ozgediz D, Roayaie K, Lee H, et al. Subcutaneous endoscopically assisted liga-tion (SEAL) of the internal ring for repair of inguinal hernias in children: report of a new technique and early results. Surg Endosc 2007;21(8):1327–31.

30. Chan KL, Tam PK. A safe laparoscopic technique for the repair of inguinal hernias in boys. J Am Coll Surg 2003;196(6):987–9.

31. Gorsler CM, Schier F. Laparoscopic herniorrhaphy in children. Surg Endosc In-terv Tech 2003;17(4):571–3.

32. Zallen G, Glick PL. Laparoscopic inversion and ligation inguinal hernia repair in girls. J Laparoendosc Adv Surg Tech 2007;17(1):143–5.

33. Yip KF, Tam PKH, Li MKW. Laparoscopic flip-flap hernioplasty: an innovative technique for pediatric hernia surgery. Surg Endosc 2004;18(7):1126–9.

34. Riquelme M, Aranda A, Riquelme-Q M. Laparoscopic pediatric inguinal hernia repair: no ligation, just resection. J Laparoendosc Adv Surg Tech 2010;20(1): 77–80.

35. Ein SH, Njere I, Ein A. Six thousand three hundred sixty-one pediatric inguinal hernias: a 35-year review. J Pediatr Surg 2006;41(5):980–6.

36. Rowe MI, Copelson LW, Clatworthy HW. The patent processus vaginalis and the inguinal hernia. J Pediatr Surg 1969;4(1):102–7.

37. Tackett LD, Breuer CK, Luks FI, et al. Incidence of contralateral inguinal hernia: a prospective analysis. J Pediatr Surg 1999;34(5):684–7 [discussion: 687–8].

38. Pellegrin K, Bensard DD, Karrer FM, et al. Laparoscopic evaluation of contralat-eral patent processus vaginalis in children. Am J Surg 1996;172(5):602–6.

39. Maillet OP, Garnier S, Dadure C, et al. Inguinal hernia in premature boys: should we systematically explore the contralateral side? J Pediatr Surg 2014;49(9): 1419–23.

40. Ballantyne A, Jawaheer G, Munro FD. Contralateral groin exploration is not justi-fied in infants with a unilateral inguinal hernia. Br J Surg 2001;88(5):720–3.

41. Marulaiah M, Atkinson J, Kukkady A, et al. Is contralateral exploration necessary in preterm infants with unilateral inguinal hernia? J Pediatr Surg 2006;41(12): 2004–7.

42. Ikeda H, Yamamoto H, Fujino J, et al. Umbilicoplasty for large protruding umbili-cus accompanying umbilical hernia: a simple and effective technique. Pediatr Surg Int 2004;20(2):105–7.

43. Shabbir J, Moore A, O'Sullivan JB, et al. Contralateral groin exploration is not justified in infants with a unilateral inguinal hernia. Ir J Med Sci 2003;172(1):18–9.

44. Clark JJ, Limm W, Wong LL. What is the likelihood of requiring contralateral inguinal hernia repair after unilateral repair? Am J Surg 2011;202(6):754–8.

45. Lee SL, Sydorak RM, Lau ST. Laparoscopic contralateral groin exploration: is it cost effective? J Pediatr Surg 2010;45(4):793–5.

46. Maddox MM, Smith DP. A long-term prospective analysis of pediatric unilateral inguinal hernias: should laparoscopy or anything else influence the management of the contralateral side? J Pediatr Urol 2008;4(2):141–5.

47. Burd RS, Heffington SH, Teague JL. The optimal approach for management of metachronous hernias in children: a decision analysis. J Pediatr Surg 2001; 36(8):1190–5.

48. Lau ST, Lee Y-H, Caty MG. Current management of hernias and hydroceles. Semin Pediatr Surg 2007;16(1):50–7.

49. Chan KWE, Lee KH, Tam YH, et al. Laparoscopic inguinal hernia repair by the hook method in emergency setting in children presenting with incarcerated inguinal hernia. J Pediatr Surg 2011;46(10):1970–3.

50. Kurkchubasche AG, Tracy TF. Inguinal hernia/hydrocele. Oper Tech Gen Surg 2004;6(4):253–68.

51. Shalaby R, Moniem Shams A, Mohamed S, et al. Two-trocar needlescopic approach to incarcerated inguinal hernia in children. J Pediatr Surg 2007;42(7): 1259–62.

52. Parelkar SV, Oak S, Bachani MK, et al. Laparoscopic repair of pediatric inguinal hernia—is vascularity of the testis at risk? A study of 125 testes. J Pediatr Surg 2011;46(9):1813–6.

53. Chan KL, Chan HY, Tam PKH. Towards a near-zero recurrence rate in laparoscopic inguinal hernia repair for pediatric patients of all ages. J Pediatr Surg 2007;42(12):1993–7.

Statement of Ownership, Management, and Circulation
(All Periodicals Publications Except Requester Publications)

UNITED STATES POSTAL SERVICE®

1. Publication Title	2. Publication Number		3. Filing Date
CLINICS IN PERINATOLOGY	001 – 744		9/18/2017

4. Issue Frequency	5. Number of Issues Published Annually	6. Annual Subscription Price
MAR, JUN, SEP, DEC	4	$299.00

7. Complete Mailing Address of Known Office of Publication (Not printer) (Street, city, county, state, and ZIP+4®)

ELSEVIER INC.
230 Park Avenue, Suite 800
New York, NY 10169

Contact Person
STEPHEN R. BUSHING

Telephone (Include area code)
215-239-3688

8. Complete Mailing Address of Headquarters or General Business Office of Publisher (Not printer)

ELSEVIER INC.
230 Park Avenue, Suite 800
New York, NY 10169

9. Full Names and Complete Mailing Addresses of Publisher, Editor, and Managing Editor (Do not leave blank)

Publisher (Name and complete mailing address)

ADRIANNE BRIGIDO, ELSEVIER INC.
1600 JOHN F KENNEDY BLVD. SUITE 1800
PHILADELPHIA, PA 19103-2899

Editor (Name and complete mailing address)

KERRY HOLLAND, ELSEVIER INC.
1600 JOHN F KENNEDY BLVD. SUITE 1800
PHILADELPHIA, PA 19103-2899

Managing Editor (Name and complete mailing address)

PATRICK MANLEY, ELSEVIER INC.
1600 JOHN F KENNEDY BLVD. SUITE 1800
PHILADELPHIA, PA 19103-2899

10. Owner (Do not leave blank. If the publication is owned by a corporation, give the name and address of the corporation immediately followed by the names and addresses of all stockholders owning or holding 1 percent or more of the total amount of stock. If not owned by a corporation, give the names and addresses of the individual owners. If owned by a partnership or other unincorporated firm, give its name and address as well as those of each individual owner. If the publication is published by a nonprofit organization, give its name and address.)

Full Name	Complete Mailing Address
WHOLLY OWNED SUBSIDIARY OF REED/ELSEVIER, US HOLDINGS	1600 JOHN F KENNEDY BLVD. SUITE 1800 PHILADELPHIA, PA 19103-2899

11. Known Bondholders, Mortgagees, and Other Security Holders Owning or Holding 1 Percent or More of Total Amount of Bonds, Mortgages, or Other Securities. If none, check box. ▶ ☐ None

Full Name	Complete Mailing Address
N/A	

12. Tax Status (For completion by nonprofit organizations authorized to mail at nonprofit rates) (Check one)
The purpose, function, and nonprofit status of this organization and the exempt status for federal income tax purposes:
☒ Has Not Changed During Preceding 12 Months
☐ Has Changed During Preceding 12 Months (Publisher must submit explanation of change with this statement)

13. Publication Title	14. Issue Date for Circulation Data Below
CLINICS IN PERINATOLOGY	JUNE 2017

15. Extent and Nature of Circulation			Average No. Copies Each Issue During Preceding 12 Months	No. Copies of Single Issue Published Nearest to Filing Date
a. Total Number of Copies (Net press run)			1020	838
b. Paid Circulation (By Mail and Outside the Mail)	(1)	Mailed Outside-County Paid Subscriptions Stated on PS Form 3541 (Include paid distribution above nominal rate, advertiser's proof copies, and exchange copies)	677	619
	(2)	Mailed In-County Paid Subscriptions Stated on PS Form 3541 (Include paid distribution above nominal rate, advertiser's proof copies, and exchange copies)	0	0
	(3)	Paid Distribution Outside the Mails Including Sales Through Dealers and Carriers, Street Vendors, Counter Sales, and Other Paid Distribution Outside USPS®	182	147
	(4)	Paid Distribution by Other Classes of Mail Through the USPS (e.g. First-Class Mail®)	0	0
c. Total Paid Distribution (Sum of 15b (1), (2), (3), and (4))		▶	859	766
d. Free or Nominal Rate Distribution (By Mail and Outside the Mail)	(1)	Free or Nominal Rate Outside-County Copies included on PS Form 3541	71	72
	(2)	Free or Nominal Rate In-County Copies Included on PS Form 3541	0	0
	(3)	Free or Nominal Rate Copies Mailed at Other Classes Through the USPS (e.g. First-Class Mail)	0	0
	(4)	Free or Nominal Rate Distribution Outside the Mail (Carriers or other means)	0	0
e. Total Free or Nominal Rate Distribution (Sum of 15d (1), (2), (3) and (4))		▶	71	72
f. Total Distribution (Sum of 15c and 15e)		▶	930	838
g. Copies not Distributed (See Instructions to Publishers #4 (page #3))		▶	90	0
h. Total (Sum of 15f and g)		▶	1020	838
i. Percent Paid (15c divided by 15f times 100)		▶	92.37%	91.41%

* If you are claiming electronic copies, go to line 16 on page 3. If you are not claiming electronic copies, skip to line 17 on page 3.

16. Electronic Copy Circulation		Average No. Copies Each Issue During Preceding 12 Months	No. Copies of Single Issue Published Nearest to Filing Date
a. Paid Electronic Copies	▶	0	0
b. Total Paid Print Copies (Line 15c) + Paid Electronic Copies (Line 16a)	▶	859	766
c. Total Print Distribution (Line 15f) + Paid Electronic Copies (Line 16a)	▶	930	838
d. Percent Paid (Both Print & Electronic Copies) (16b divided by 16c × 100)	▶	92.37%	91.41%

☒ I certify that 50% of all my distributed copies (electronic and print) are paid above a nominal price.

17. Publication of Statement of Ownership

☒ If the publication is a general publication, publication of this statement is required. Will be printed in the DECEMBER 2017 issue of this publication. ☐ Publication not required.

18. Signature and Title of Editor, Publisher, Business Manager, or Owner

STEPHEN R. BUSHING - INVENTORY DISTRIBUTION CONTROL MANAGER

Date 9/18/2017

I certify that all information furnished on this form is true and complete. I understand that anyone who furnishes false or misleading information on this form or who omits material or information requested on the form may be subject to criminal sanctions (including fines and imprisonment) and/or civil sanctions (including civil penalties).

PS Form 3526, July 2014 [Page 3 of 4 (see instructions page 4)] PSN: 7530-01-000-9931 PRIVACY NOTICE: See our privacy policy on www.usps.com

PS Form 3526, July 2014 (Page 1 of 4 (see instructions page 4)) PSN 7530-01-000-9931 PRIVACY NOTICE: See our privacy policy on www.usps.com

Moving?

Make sure your subscription moves with you!

To notify us of your new address, find your **Clinics Account Number** (located on your mailing label above your name), and contact customer service at:

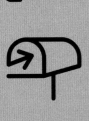

Email: journalscustomerservice-usa@elsevier.com

800-654-2452 (subscribers in the U.S. & Canada)
314-447-8871 (subscribers outside of the U.S. & Canada)

Fax number: 314-447-8029

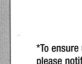

Elsevier Health Sciences Division
Subscription Customer Service
3251 Riverport Lane
Maryland Heights, MO 63043

*To ensure uninterrupted delivery of your subscription, please notify us at least 4 weeks in advance of move.

ELSEVIER

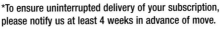